Creative Teaching Strategies for the
Nurse Educator

Creative Teaching Strategies for the Nurse Educator

Judith W. Herrman, PhD, RN
Assistant Professor
University of Delaware
Newark, Delaware

F. A. DAVIS COMPANY • Philadelphia

F. A. Davis Company
1915 Arch Street
Philadelphia, PA 19103
www.fadavis.com

Printed in the United States of America

Last digit indicates print number: 10 9 8 7 6 5 4 3

Publisher, Nursing: Joanne P. DaCunha, RN, MSN
Director of Content Development: Darlene D. Pedersen, RN, MSN
Developmental Editor: Anne-Adele Wight
Project Editor: Padraic Maroney
Art and Design Manager: Carolyn O'Brien

As new scientific information becomes available through basic and clinical research, recommended treatments and drug therapies undergo changes. The author(s) and publisher have done everything possible to make this book accurate, up to date, and in accord with accepted standards at the time of publication. The author(s), editors, and publisher are not responsible for errors or omissions or for consequences from application of the book, and make no warranty, expressed or implied, in regard to the contents of the book. Any practice described in this book should be applied by the reader in accordance with professional standards of care used in regard to the unique circumstances that may apply in each situation. The reader is advised always to check product information (package inserts) for changes and new information regarding dose and contraindications before administering any drug. Caution is especially urged when using new or infrequently ordered drugs.

Library of Congress Cataloging-in-Publication Data

Herrman, Judith W.
    Creative teaching strategies for the nurse educator / Judith W. Herrman.
    p. ; cm.
    Includes bibliographical references and index.

    ISBN-13: 978-0-8036-1432-1
    ISBN-10: 0-8036-1432-2

    1. Nursing—Study and teaching. 2. Creative teaching. I. Title.
    [DNLM: 1. Education, Nursing—methods. 2. Teaching—methods. WY 18 H551c 2008]
    RT71.H47 2008
    610.73071'1—dc22

    2007028821

Reviewers

Betsy Frank, PhD, RN
Professor
Indiana State University
Terre Haute, Indiana

Savina Schoenhofer, PhD, RN
Professor
Alcorn State University
Natchez, Missouri

Roz Seymour, EdD, RN
Professor Emeritus
East Tennessee State University
Johnson City, Tennessee

Nancy Sharts-Hopko, PhD, RN, FAAN
Professor and Director, Doctoral Program
Villanova, University
Villanova, Pennsylvania

Esperanza Villenueva Joyce, EdD. CNS, RN
Assistant Vice President of Nursing Education and Director SON
Ohio University
Athens, Ohio

Acknowledgments

Whenever a task comes to a close one considers all those who helped make the project happen. For this initiative the list is long! I would like to thank Joanne DaCunha and those at F.A. Davis for their support and guidance. I would like to offer sincere thanks to my talented colleagues who inspired many of the strategies in this text. Years of teaching classes and working with creative and energetic nurses and nurse educators have offered many potential innovative teaching methods and a created a sincere desire to connect with students. This book reflects the talent and dedication inherent of nursing educators both in academic and practice settings.

Finally, I would like to extend the greatest level of appreciation to my husband, my three sons, my parents, my friends, and my family. Their devotion, support, and love will continue to add meaning to my life and motivate me to continue to grow in my personal and professional endeavors.

Judith W. Herrman, PhD, RN

Contents

3   Strategies for Large Classrooms 53

"The mediocre teacher tells. The good teacher explains. The superior teacher demonstrates. The great teacher inspires." —William Arthur Ward

Challenges 53

Ideas 54

4   Strategies for Small Classes 97

"Implementing creative teaching strategies that will change a classroom from a four walled room with educational hopes into an environment that is infused with excitement, curiosity, and genuine student learning." —Simplicio

Challenges 97

Ideas 98

5 Strategies for Clinical Instruction and Orientation 157

"I take one minute a few times a day to look at my goals and see what I want to learn . . . . I can teach myself what I want to learn more easily by taking one minute to catch myself doing something right. . . . We are at our best when we teach ourselves what we need to learn." —Johnson and Johnson

Challenges 157

Ideas 158

6   Strategies for Discussion Groups 207

"Shared perspectives, shared knowledge, and shared experiences are the key foundational building blocks of creativity." —Simplicio

Challenges 207

Ideas 208

7   Strategies for Teaching Research 259

"Education is not the filling of a pail, but the lighting of a fire." — William Butler Yeats *"The highest result of education is tolerance."* — Helen Keller

8   Conclusion 285

"Teaching was the hardest work I have ever done, and it remains the hardest work I have done to date." —Ann Richards

Annotated Bibliography 295

Strategy Locator 314

Index 319

Chapter 1
The Art of Innovation

"The art of teaching is the art of assisting discovery."—Mark Van Doran

WHAT IS AN INNOVATION?

To examine creative teaching strategies clearly, we must define innovation and its relationship to teaching. Schell[1] defines innovation as the use of nontraditional methods in learning settings. In essence, an innovation is any educational strategy not usually performed by the instructor or witnessed previously by a class.

Nowhere does this definition mention the extent or degree of creativity. Therefore the innovation doesn't have to be major; any deviation, large or small, from custom is considered an innovation. Anything you haven't done before or don't usually do can fall within this category. It's important to remember that any strategy new to the students is considered an innovation even if it isn't new to you. Finally, the innovation lies not only in the teaching strategy, but in the method the individual nurse educator uses to present it.

Schell[1] believes that innovative methods meet the needs of today's nurses and nursing students. New methods can and should be used to enhance learning for nurses and to educate nursing students. Innovative strategies provide a foundation from which to design classroom activities, assignments, approaches to content, new ways to teach previously taught material, and evaluation methods. New nurse educators may find these creative methods helpful in developing their own teaching style. Instructors who have taught for several years, or who have taught the same material several times, may appreciate the need for novel, creative, and objective-driven strategies.

HOW DO INNOVATIVE STRATEGIES ENHANCE LEARNING?

Enjoyment and Inspiration

According to Tanner[2], nursing educators must assess and potentially change the way they teach. Student populations have become more diverse, and public expectations and health-care demands have changed. Many nurse educators teach the way they were taught. For some of us that's a recent experience; for others, more remote history.

Significantly, we remember the learning experiences we found most powerful. We retain information that was delivered in an unique, innovative, and enjoyable way. Perhaps most important, we chose to teach because we believe that these positive and negative learning experiences, information gathered throughout our practice, and a desire to "pass it on" are key in the teaching-learning process.

Differences in learning styles warrant new and different ways to interact with students and promote learning. Many nurse educators practice their craft year after year. There's a saying, "Anyone can face a crisis—it's the day-to-day living that wears you out." Teaching on a one-time basis to a crowd of excited learners may require a different level of creativity and innovation than a routine teaching session or a class that teaches less popular material. It's in the more routine situation that creative teaching strategies really earn their merit. Innovations slipped into current teaching methods can provide a diversion and reinforce material that might otherwise be forgotten.

Not only are today's learners different from those of previous generations—so are their expectations of the learning experience. Today's students are consumers with high standards for teachers, sometimes presenting a challenge to even the most accomplished and seasoned instructors. By increasing the level of enjoyment in learning, creative teaching strategies can inspire students to attend class, prepare for class, and maintain vigilance during the session.

No Lecture Bashing Here

I wrote this book from a belief that the time-honored method of teaching—the lecture—is effective, efficient, and meets the needs of most learners. Oermann[3] states that lecturing is time efficient, especially with larger classes, and that most nurse educators are comfortable with this technique. The lecture as a teaching method has come under a lot of fire lately. Many now consider it passive, traditionalist, and less in tune with the needs of current learners.

Woodring[4] comments that nursing education literature has taken to "lecture-bashing." This book does not "lecture-bash." Instead it recommends interspersing creative strategies with tried-and-true lecture methods as a way to enhance active learning and retention. Often educators are charged with assuming new teaching methods that "throw the baby out with the bath water." Teachers are told of great disservices imposed by traditional ways of teaching and are urged to make huge changes in their methods. The nurse educator of today probably doesn't have time to overhaul teaching methods or to update previously taught materials to a new method of instruction.

The strategies discussed in this book are presented as short, purposeful innovations meant to complement and reinforce lecture material. Attention spans have changed, students are more stressed, and teaching now uses a variety of media. We must consider innovative methods that break into traditional content, yet still allow us to cover material and meet class objectives. In essence, the lecture method presents information effectively; creative strategies provide diversions that reinforce key material or areas of emphasis. These strategies are grounded in the belief that students are more likely to remember content presented in an atmosphere of creative learning and fun.

You can use innovative teaching methods to highlight key points of a class. This method helps to focus the content, allowing students to sort out information and establish priorities. Setting priorities is always a challenge in nursing education and practice alike. Using an innovative strategy to highlight selected content helps students to hone in on vital information.

Another challenge of nursing school teaching may be summarized in the statement, "We keep adding content to nursing education and don't take anything out—we just talk faster." This sentence reflects our need to differentiate the "need to know" from the "nice to know." A creative teaching strategy can put the "need to know" label where it needs to go.

What Are the Barriers to Innovative Teaching?

Now we've discussed all the reasons to introduce creative teaching strategies. It's time to address some of the barriers that teachers encounter when attempting to weave creative strategies throughout their material. Schell[1] identifies the barriers to innovative teaching as perceived self-worth, social support and authority, tradition, physical environment, past educational experiences, time, and communication skills.

Never Enough Time

Years of teaching and presenting this material to nurse educators has distilled the barriers down to a few categories. The most formidable perceived barrier is time. It takes time to prepare a strategy: the instructor has to relate it to class material, assemble equipment, and practice a smooth transition so that the strategy will fit naturally into the class. In addition, class time may be limited, and creative strategies leave less time for traditional methods.

Nursing educators feel the need to cover content. We all think, "If I don't say it, they won't learn it, and it will be my fault." Instead, we should be thinking of ways to use valuable classroom time to clarify concepts, reinforce more difficult elements, and synthesize other learning methods. Such methods may include assignments, readings, and hands-on experience. By changing our mind-set about the goals of the classroom, we can better incorporate creative strategies despite limited time.

I say "perceived barrier" because these strategies don't take as much time as you might think. You need time to think of, plan, and prepare each strategy, but once it's developed, it can be adapted for several class contexts. In a section of Chapter 8, entitled *Finding the Teaching Fuel,* we discuss sources of material for developing a toolbox of adaptable creative strategies. We should also borrow strategies from other successful nurse educators and share effective methods with fellow teachers.

Out on a Limb

Another, more subtle, barrier is self-confidence. Creative teaching strategies include an element of risk. Instructors may need to step out of their usual role, or perhaps convey a different image than usual. Some strategies may "crash and burn," not meeting the students' needs, not working well with a particular group, or failing in some other way.

Don't worry—you can mold creative strategies to your specific teaching style and comfort level. You may need to stretch outside your usual classroom techniques, but you should never feel uncomfortable or awkward. A good rule of thumb is that if you feel uncomfortable, the students will too, negating the value of the teaching strategy. You'll need to prepare in advance and be comfortable with your strategy; it should flow smoothly, fit well with the class objectives, and not interrupt learning.

A key point: you, the instructor, must understand and feel comfortable with the material. You need clinical experience with the content, familiarity with your lecture material, and a clear idea of your learning objectives and teaching goals for the session. The first time you teach a topic, use only one or two creative strategies to drive home points—holding back a little will ensure that you deliver the content. As you start covering the same material repeatedly or in greater depth, you can get more creative with your strategies and feel more confident that the information is getting across. It's especially important to remember that in today's teaching environment, faculty must frequently teach varied topics, may teach outside their own skills or specialty, and be given the opportunity to teach on a repetitive basis.

Culture Versus Creativity

The final barrier may be the teaching culture of the institution. A school or service agency with a traditional culture may not accept new or innovative strategies. The administration may adhere to certain teaching habits or may simply not see the value of creativity in teaching. Individual instructors may need to confront this issue and teach in the way they believe will best serve the students. Teaching cultures are clearly changing. By developing individual teaching styles, instructors can support institutions as they begin to embrace innovation.

We could go on brainstorming to find more barriers, but instead, let's focus on the reasons you can and should use innovations in your teaching.

WHAT KIND OF INSTRUCTOR ARE YOU?

Assess Your Teaching Style

An important foundation for creative teaching strategies is an honest and accurate assessment of personal teaching style, ability, and knowledge level. Often instructors are hired or delegated to teach because of their ability to speak in public. Although public speaking is an important skill, building a teaching environment that encourages learning requires much more. To make a significant impact, teachers must take a comprehensive, holistic approach. This is where self-assessment and creative teaching strategies enter the picture.

Sometimes self-assessment is as simple as asking yourself, "Why do I teach?" By analyzing their personal attraction to teaching while assessing their strengths and weaknesses, instructors may begin to explore personal teaching philosophies and styles. Self-assessment can overcome some of the previously mentioned challenges of infusing creativity into the classroom.

Identify Your Strengths

Some factors to assess are previous experience with teaching, clinical experience with certain populations, and interpersonal skills. Teachers may take on the roles of sage, mentor, information juggler, expert, colleague, and entertainer—nursing instructors often feel like all these characters at different times. The following questions can help you to assess your teaching as well as to set personal goals:

- Are you comfortable enough with the material to deliver it in an understandable manner?
- Do you have enough expertise with the subject matter to provide a personal perspective? If not, can you glean the more subtle aspects

from reading, talking with others, or capitalizing on the experience levels of class participants?

- Do you have the talent to create a learning environment in which students feel free to ask questions, clarify material, and consider alternatives?
- Can you use feedback and evaluative information to give students a clear picture of their progress in the class and to help them improve understanding and performance?
- Do you present a positive role model for the profession and for the need for lifelong learning?
- Do you foster cooperation among students, encourage active learning, and communicate high expectations?
- Do you respect divergent learning styles and adapt teaching to meet the needs of various learners in the group?
- Do you organize your presentations, class conduct, and class structure? Although some teachers are more organized than others, new students need structured methods. These give them a foundation on which to learn, organize their own thoughts, and pattern concepts so that they make sense.
- Do you feel comfortable presenting material in varying settings and with different-sized groups? Can you adapt your teaching methods and styles in these circumstances to provide the greatest benefits for the class?
- Do you have the energy to teach with enthusiasm?

The Student's-eye View

It's also important to consider what each class expects from the teachers. In Schell's study[1], students said that they wanted their teachers to:

- Be caring and promote personal growth.
- Include creativity and a variety of strategies in their teaching.
- Be willing to learn as well as teach, demonstrating approachability and availability, and fostering an interactive environment.
- Maintain teacher-student boundaries.
- Demonstrate respect for others and personal qualities deserving of respect.
- Provide feedback to their students.

These statements provide an acceptable consensus on what students perceive as the qualities needed for success. Next we'll consider the ways in which instructors and students can combine their personal styles with creative teaching strategies for the best possible result.

WHO ARE NEW LEARNERS AND HOW DO THEY LEARN?

Know Your Students

In a learning situation, responsibility lies on both sides. One of the educator's responsibilities is to assess the students and develop strategies aimed at their individual and collective needs.

Several methods can be used to describe today's learners and their own specific learning needs. First, as with any cohort, we must remember that they are a heterogeneous lot, reflecting different ages, cultural backgrounds, contexts, beliefs, and learning styles. Today's groups of nursing students may be more diverse than ever before. In fact, their heterogeneity may create the greatest need for innovative teaching strategies. A participative lecture interspersed with creative strategies, rather than a straight lecture format, may attend to a greater number of learning styles and needs.

Are Today's Learners Different?

One characteristic of many present-day learners is the need to have fun, in essence, to be entertained while learning. This is not to say that creative teaching strategies should "dumb down" the lesson or make it less meaningful. However, a generation that has been entertained with rapid-fire stimulation may need increased impetus to pay attention to class content, especially if it's delivered in a dry manner. This type of learner benefits from strategies to enhance retention and enjoyment in the classroom.

Conversely, many of today's learners catch on to concepts more quickly than previous generations did, increasing the likelihood that they may lose interest in boring or repetitive material. It is not enough to provide keen insights and experiences to augment material. Today's learners expect the material to be enjoyable and perhaps intriguing. On the other hand, other students in the class many learn at a more traditional pace, adding to the challenge for teachers.

Although creative strategies don't guarantee fascination, they may provide diversion and enjoyable breaks in the rhythm of class. Marketers tell us that the television viewer's attention span approximates 6 to 10 minutes.

This statistic is reflected in the current interval between commercials during television shows. Therefore, methods paced to the prevailing attention span of the class may be the most effective in reinforcing material and keeping students attentive.

Sensory Learning

Also important are the categories of learning styles: visual, auditory, and kinesthetic. Do your students learn predominantly by sight, hearing, or feeling and touching? Different learning styles warrant varying teaching strategies. In the general population, 80 percent of learners are thought to be visual, 10 percent auditory, and 10 percent kinesthetic.

Many contend that nurses have a greater propensity toward kinesthetic learning, or learning by feel, demonstration, or manipulation. This idea is no surprise to teachers of psychomotor skills, in which demonstrating, touching, practicing, and proving competency are the most effective ways to achieve mastery. Learners who can identify their style may also discover the study methods that will best enhance their learning.

Innovative strategies that allow for the greatest sensory stimulation may be the most effective. Several of these strategies capture more than one sense, allowing divergent learners to assimilate information on their own personal level. For example, showing a film clip in class may appeal to visual and auditory learners, whereas using dime-store prizes appropriate to content may help kinesthetic and visual learners remember material.

Hemisphere Dominance

Other authors have recommended analyzing brain dominance in the learner to evaluate learning styles. Left-brain dominant people are analytical and detail oriented; right-brain dominant people are more global and creative in their learning styles. The need to adapt teaching styles to both left- and right-brain dominant individuals is a key responsibility of teachers. The left-brain learner may be resistant to creative teaching strategies, seeing them as trivial. The right-brain learner may need focus on objectives to ensure that the teaching strategy is valuable and goal directed, rather than merely fun.

Remembering that each of us uses both brain hemispheres is essential to the enhancement of learning. Assessing your class for a predominant "brain side" may help you create effective, well-received class strategies.

When Were They Young?

Finally, we must consider generational differences when assessing learners. Chester[5] notes that in identifying generational differences and determining teaching applications, "The question is not, 'How old are you?', but, 'When were you young?'" Asking students to remember whether their experiences in grade school were dominated by a blackboard or a computer screen may offer insights into their current learning needs. Young people who are used to the computer, television, and newer technologies learn at a rapid pace. This indoctrination causes learners to demand interesting, relevant content.

Recent studies focus on generational thinking and the impact of generational differences on education, interests, and performance in the workplace. Several newly available resources delineate generations according to common learning characteristics[6] (see also the Annotated Bibliography).

The Veterans

Traditionalists, or "Veterans," born between 1922 and 1945, tend to be attentive, respectful, and passive learners. They respond to more traditional lecture methods and usually are motivated to learn and work. According to Hobbs,[7] the Veterans build on previous wisdom, respect wisdom in others, and learn best when respected for their current levels of knowledge and experience.

This group tends to find creative strategies the most unpleasant. They want to stay in their comfort zone, the lecture format, and their ideals of traditional teacher-student roles. They also may resist group work. In contrast, they tend to follow orders or directives in the classroom. This tendency may result in their cooperation, albeit reluctant, with creative strategies.

The Baby Boomers

The "Baby Boomers," born between 1946 and 1964—now both students and the parents of students—have come to realize their role as the largest generation of consumers. Both demanding and accepting, this group may or may not endorse technology but has high standards for teaching. Boomers frequently place the responsibility for learning on the quality of the teaching. They will also devote considerable effort to learning if they perceive the information to be valid, relevant, and ultimately useful in their future life or work.

The Boomers learn from experience. They want to be respected for their current levels of experience and learn best with experiential teaching strategies.

Generation X

Those born between 1965 and 1980, sometimes known as "Generation X-ers," respond well to creativity in learning and teaching methods. This group finds the innovations associated with technology and health care intriguing and a challenge, rather than an obstacle. They are a group who enjoy learning but for whom learning needs to be enjoyable. This generation does not remember life without a television and were adolescents during the onset of the computer age. They see education as a necessary step toward another goal, and they work toward achieving a balance between work and play.

Generation Why?

The final group, termed "Millennials," or "Generation Why?", are the "twenty-somethings." They represent the bulk of nursing students and nurses just entering the workforce, who require orientation and intensive educational interventions. This group learns at a rapid pace, is comfortable with innovation, expects learning to have a creative side, and advocates for their own learning needs. Generation Why? learns and lives at one with technology and generally embraces group work because of indoctrination in group methods throughout their education.

Would You Enjoy Your Class?

All of these learning characteristics—whether heterogeneously oriented, culturally based, influenced by brain dominance, or responding to the unique characteristics of a generation—can be distilled to a common concept: respect for the learner. The educator who responds to the needs of the student, assesses groups for learning needs and styles, and demonstrates a sincere attitude of caring and desire to teach will have the greatest success with innovative teaching strategies. A quotation helps to summarize this material: "If you had you for a teacher, would you enjoy coming to class?"[5]

HOW CAN YOU USE THIS BOOK?

The ultimate goal of this book is to increase learning and retention making teaching more enjoyable and effective. For many of us who t nursing students or nurses, our goals are to enhance critical thinl encourage team work, foster a sense of lifelong learning, facilitate lem solving, and stimulate active learning. In the end, we hop meeting our goals will increase the workforce of intelligent, skille high-quality nurses.

You can use this book in any way you choose. Whether you use an isolated creative strategy in your teaching repertoire or decide to create a more substantial revision in your teaching style, this book is here to help you. That being said, here are a few suggestions to assist you in using it:

- Feel free to use your own creativity and teaching needs to mold the teaching strategies. Your own style and content may dictate adaptation. For example, you may need to change a strategy to fit the room setup. Or, as you "read" your class, you may sense that a strategy as planned will not work with this group. Mold each strategy as you find necessary.

  The creativity I hope to inspire includes the ability to revise strategies to best meet your needs. Use the *Personal Journal Pages* at the end of each chapter to note how a strategy was used, what worked and what didn't, and potential uses of the strategy in the future. As you read this book at your leisure, should you have any, use the *Personal Journal Pages* to make notes about your possible use of the strategies and add your own comments. This interactive feature of the book will add to its usefulness and your personal application of material.

- Strategies in specific chapters may easily be transferred to other teaching venues. For instance, a strategy discussed in the clinical teaching chapter may be revised for use in a large or small classroom. The strategies in this text were chosen on the basis of their previous success; it's up to you to determine their usefulness elsewhere and modify them as you need to.

- To avoid "creativity fatigue," make sure you use creative teaching strategies appropriately and in small doses. Suddenly incorporating 20 strategies in an hour-long class will not only exhaust and frustrate the class, thereby hampering learning, but will also steer you away from your objectives. Instead, use one or two strategies per class to emphasize key points, provide transition, or break up difficult material.

- Remember that these strategies are designed to be interspersed with your customary teaching styles and methods. They are not intended to replace current methods or to demand a total overhaul of your teaching.

- Staff development educators probably need no reminder that nurses are tired and overworked. Creative strategies that are fun and contribute to a collaborative learning atmosphere will help the students pay attention and remember the material. Generational differences may be even more pronounced in the workplace than

in academic settings, increasing your need to attend to a variety of learning styles and customs.

Nurses who work long hours feel pulled from their client care priorities and demand incentives to pay attention to new concepts. In addition, nurses may perceive educational days in the practice setting as time off. Innovative teaching strategies may help center nurses on class priorities and provide an incentive for learning and application to practice.

- I invented many strategies as the need arose during active teaching of nurses in academic and practice sessions. I experienced other strategies as a student in nursing continuing education classes and derived still others from fellow nurse educators. The importance of sharing for the common good, while giving credit to developers of strategies if they are known, is key to the enhancement of nursing education. A Web site has been created to capitalize on the creativity of many people and create a resource that will keep growing. The link is http://davisplus. fadavis.com/herrman. Please share your successes, challenges, new ideas, and questions on this Web site for the benefit of all! Most important, have fun with this book. Pick it up and put it down whenever you want to. You may choose to read it cover to cover or peruse it like a phone book to find what you need. The *Personal Journal Pages* will help you meet your own teaching needs. Their focus is on helping you enjoy the strategies, incorporate them into your personal teaching, and evaluate their future use. If you can create an environment that promotes sharing, mutual respect, and active learning—an atmosphere that establishes rapport with each student—you will have a positive impact on the learning experience of your class. Enjoy!

References

1. Schell, K: The process of innovative teaching in the generic baccalaureate nursing classroom: A cross-case analysis. Unpublished doctoral dissertation, Widener University, 2001.
2. Tanner, CA: Innovations in nursing education. Journal of Nursing Education 36(6): 243, 1997.
3. Oermann, MH: Using active learning in lecture: Best of "both worlds." International Journal of Nursing Education Scholarship 1(1): 1–9, 2004.
4. Woodring, BC: Lecture is not a four-letter word! In Fuszard, B: Innovative Teaching Strategies in Nursing. Aspen, Gaithersburg, MD, 1995.
5. Chester, E: A Quick Look at Generation Why. Accessed on January 10, 2007 from www.generationwhy.com.

6. Hopkins, M, and Merilatt, J: Bridging the generation gap. ModRN, pp 56–60, Fall, 2006.
7. Hobbs, J: Generations: A walk through the past, present, and future of nursing. Public presentation, Sigma Theta Tau International Convention, Indianapolis, 2005.

Personal Journal Pages

Getting Started with Icebreakers

"In the first minutes, you set the stage ... you orchestrate how they talk to each other." —Michele Deck

Challenges

- Classes in which the students don't know each other may take on an impersonal quality.
- If you don't know the students, they may be difficult to teach, lacking a sense of community and mutual learning.
- If the students don't know you, the class may lack the level of trust required to allow creative teaching strategies to flourish.
- You as the instructor have the responsibility to set the stage for learning—it's efficient to simply jump in, but you may miss a great opportunity for team building and creating an active learning environment.
- Creative teaching strategies may surprise some learners and therefore may be met with resistance.
- Participants may enter a class with disparate expectations and motivations for learning.
- Participants may be reluctant to talk within a class.
- Whether a class is a one-time event or an ongoing experience, students may be less comfortable in a formal learning environment. Effective, entertaining icebreakers may warm them up.
- You may need to "read" the dynamic of your class to determine their responsiveness to interactive or more personal types of icebreakers.

Using introductions and icebreakers helps set the tone for the class and provides a forum for the creative teaching focus. You're getting the class on the right wavelength for innovative teaching and learning methods. These strategies also give you an opportunity to quickly assess the students; you can discover their levels of motivation, backgrounds, objectives for the class, and openness to innovative teaching strategies. Icebreakers may initiate conversation, allowing for future participation and group discussion. Most important, they provide a means for the instructor to build a rapport with the class and to ensure that both you and the students are comfortable and ready for learning.

IDEAS

Shapes Define Your Personality

General Description   This strategy displays shapes on an overhead projector, in PowerPoint™ format, or as regular slides. Participants choose a shape on the basis of selected criteria, and then discussion ensues.

Preparation and Equipment   You'll need an overhead projector, blackboard, PowerPoint setup, and writing implements. You may draw the pictures in front of the class or bring them already prepared.

Example of the Strategy at Work   To break the ice, participants are asked to determine which shape matches their style of nursing, personality, learning style, or any other personal characteristic (Fig. 2–1). As an additional icebreaker, encourage class members not to pick shapes that resemble their body types. The instructor then explains the psychogeometric interpretations of each shape. Psychogeometric theory, according to Dellinger,[1] dictates that the following shape choices appear to correlate with certain personality types.

- Squares: Organized, structured, rigid, task-oriented, concrete, no ideas—all "do"
- Circles: People lovers—caring, nurturing, harmonious
- Rectangles: In transition—confused, don't know what to choose
- Triangles: Leaders—make decisions, work well with squares, take charge, delegate, may be ruthless in their leadership styles and management methods
- "Squiggly" line: Creative, relaxed, idea people—little work, few results

Participants should be given the choice of whether or not to divulge their shape in class.

ICEBREAKER EXAMPLE:

Which shape best describes you as a nurse?

Team building...

Fig. 2–1.   Which shape best describes you as a nurse?

The instructor should "read" the class to determine whether this disclosure would encourage group dynamics.

Ideas for Use

- This strategy provides unique insights into the group, individual personalities, and how each individual relates and contributes to group functioning.
- Simply by knowing the group better, students may become more comfortable and ready to participate.
- **Shapes Define Your Personality** may provoke some self-exploration into priorities, thoughts, and abilities.
- This strategy makes a good team-building exercise. After students select their shapes, the class can discuss how the shapes may be used to diagnose group strengths and weaknesses. A group of

triangles—all leaders—may have a difficult time reaching consensus. A group of squiggly lines might never produce results, but would be very creative.

- As discussion continues, members are able to appreciate the valuable role each shape brings to the group process, and to understand that a diversity of talents and ideas is needed to optimize group functioning.
- This strategy is great for building a collegial spirit in a clinical or orientation group.

Get In Line

General Description   This strategy is great for the first day of class or for a 1-day class. It's especially useful for classes in which students will be asked to participate actively or to work in groups, or when students appear rooted in their seats and not engaged in the learning process. The strategy is limited to a group of approximately 10 to 20, although larger groups may be divided.

In this exercise, students line up according to age, birth month, number of years in a position or with an agency, or alphabetically by first or last name. The fun in this exercise is that the students are forbidden to talk or write. They must use nonverbal communication, such as lip synching, hand gestures, and facial expressions, to determine the correct order.

Preparation and Equipment   No preparation or equipment is required. The efficacy of this exercise may be limited by the size of the room.

Example of the Strategy at Work   At the beginning of the semester I have used this exercise to get students up, active, and acquainted with each other. Quiet or nonparticipative students may become more comfortable after having this opportunity to interact with others.

Ideas for Use

- If the class is large enough to divide into several groups, each group may try to finish the task first, adding the element of competition.
- This strategy exemplifies the value of nonverbal communication, the frustration of being unable to talk, and the difficulties of being unable to understand the dominant language spoken in a particular setting.
- The group finishing first may be offered a prize.
- Classes may be asked to develop their own ideas for the order of the line.

Introduce Each Other

General Description   This strategy is just what the title states: the class members pair up, talk for a designated period, and then are asked to **Introduce Each Other** to the class at large. Pairs may be given a discussion topic, such as "What is your name?," "Why are you taking this class?," "What type of nursing do you do (want to do)?," "What's the most significant aspect of your life?," or "What was the most significant event in your life?"

Preparation and Equipment   No equipment or preparation is required. This strategy is most feasible with groups of about 20.

Example of the Strategy at Work   This initiative is most successful if all groups have the chance to **Introduce Each Other,** so you must allow adequate time. The most valuable time to use this exercise is at the beginning of a class session, when group comfort is being established. You can ask the class to **Introduce Each Other** to their neighbors or ask them to get up and move to another part of the room.

Ideas for Use

- The strategy may be limited to an introduction within each pair of students. This version omits the need for students to **Introduce Each Other** to the larger group. It is valuable in larger classes or when the available time is restricted. Some classes prefer this version of the strategy because it's less obtrusive.

- Introductions may assist in breaking up cliques or forging new relationships within a class. You can set a ground rule requiring participants to pair up with someone they don't know.

- Use this strategy to combat the after-lunch "sleepies" or with a characteristically nonparticipative class.

- Introduction questions may be tailored to meet specific needs, determined by the objectives of the class. For example, you can ask a nursing education class to discuss educational challenges, the most creative strategies used, or the most embarrassing teaching moment. Any of these subjects will incite discussions. As you use this strategy, you may stumble on questions that are both fun and relevant to your teaching topics.

- A great way to use **Introduce Each Other** is to have students pair up. They stand face to face and observe each other for several seconds. Each person then turns around and makes three changes in his or her appearance: removing glasses, changing jewelry or hairstyle, moving clothing around, or altering position in some way. The pair then turns back around, and each tries to identify the changes in the other. This tactic reinforces the observation skills needed in nursing and assessment.

This exercise can also stimulate creativity: the pairs of students can repeat it to see how many changes they and their partners can undergo. The pairs then **Introduce Each Other** and discuss the changes. Not only does the strategy focus on assessment and creative problem-solving, it gets students up and moving. This version is fun and works well in large classes.

A Brush with Fame

My colleague Michele Deck uses an innovative icebreaker to work with groups of various sizes and compositions. She calls it **A Brush with Fame.** In this strategy, students pair up and share their experiences of meeting a famous person. Deck has found that this exercise provides just the right balance between personal information and privacy. To illustrate the need for privacy in health care, she emphasizes the need to keep professional **Brushes with Fame** confidential, although they can be shared freely in personal life. She tells the amusing story of a class participant who won over the class by going on a double date with a famous rock star. Pairs can share their **Brushes with Fame** and develop a rapport with the whole class by selecting one **Brush** that's particularly special.

"Why Are You in Nursing?" and Other Mysteries

General Description   As in the previous strategy, class members form groups of two or three and explore a question posed by the instructor. Pairs or trios may or may not be asked to report the results to the group. Questions may be general or may be specific to the class content or objectives. This strategy can facilitate active listening and active learning and loosen up the class.

Preparation and Equipment   You can print the questions and directions for the activity on a PowerPoint or regular slide, or may simply ask the question or questions out loud.

Example of the Strategy at Work   I've found that this strategy works best when students are given a focused amount of time (5 minutes) and are asked to list a specific number of items. In the exercise shown (Box 2–1), done at the beginning of a pharmacology course, students are asked to come up with five reasons why nurses need to know pharmacology. Then the group shares their ideas. Rather than accept a list of reasons from the instructor, students become more invested in the topic by contributing their own ideas and discussions.

Box 2–1.
Why Do Nurses Need to Learn Pharmacology?

Why must nurses learn about medications: their actions, their uses, and their nursing implications?
- Think about the question.
- Talk about it with your neighbor.
- What five reasons did you come up with?
- Share your thoughts with the class.

Ideas for Use

- Consider this strategy any time you plan to teach a list of ideas.
- New nursing students or new graduates may be asked, "Why are you in nursing?," "Why did you pick this agency?," and "Why is it important for nurses to know about _____?"
- For continuing education, you'll need to ask, "Why is it important that nurses know ACLS?," "Why is it important for nurses to know the legal aspects of nursing practice?," or any other question that relates to the class objectives.
- **"Why Are You in Nursing?"** can be used at the end of a class to review key concepts, do a mini-evaluation of learning, or open up the floor for questions. Students are asked, "How do you think the information in this class will enhance your nursing practice?" and discussion follows.
- This strategy may be done in pairs or trios.
- **"Why Are You in Nursing?"** can set the stage for further participation in class, whether the students answer your questions about difficult material or formulate their own questions.
- You can ask the same questions without dividing the class into small groups. Be aware that only certain people tend to participate in class. Those who don't generally participate are allowed to remain passive during this version of the exercise. The questions do, however, set the stage for later questions that may be put to the class. At that time, you should encourage the quiet students to speak up.

Let's Discuss

General Description   To set students at ease, you may want to begin class with an informal, conversational tone. This will entice learners to listen more attentively. Facial expressions may cue the instructor to the timing of this and other strategies.

By building collegiality, **Let's Discuss** develops rapport among the students. In this method, the instructor stimulates discussion by saying, **"Let's Discuss** your past experiences with_____ ," "**Let's Discuss** this material: _____ ," or, "**Let's Discuss** the meaning of _____ in nursing practice." This method tells your class that you appreciate their knowledge levels and their experience. It also allows students to understand that not all experiences are positive, and may introduce some ways of dealing with negative encounters.

Preparation and Equipment   No preparation or equipment is required for this strategy.

Example of the Strategy at Work   This method has been used many times with a variety of topics. By simply posing a question, you urge students to share their experiences. You might begin an infant resuscitation class with "**Let's Discuss** your previous experiences with neonatal resuscitation." This strategy guides a preliminary discussion of the issue, clarifies what the class knows, and identifies any misconceptions. Other topics have included "**Let's Discuss** your previous experience with diabetes," "**Let's Discuss** your previous experiences with nurses," "**Let's Discuss** your previous experiences with cross-training," "**Let's Discuss** how you were able to learn about a new procedure or piece of equipment," and "**Let's Discuss** your previous experiences with cancer." A cautionary note: **Let's Discuss** requires students to participate. Your role is to judge the success of the strategy by determining whether you can get students to talk. Part of the value of this strategy is to highlight complex concepts that students don't find particularly relevant. For example, in a community nursing course, the topic was the value of community assessment. Several community assessment charts and criteria were scanned into PowerPoint and shown to the class. Conversation began with "**Let's Discuss** where you grew up." Students described their neighborhoods and compared them with those they might work in during clinical rotations. In this situation, community assessment was made real through a discussion about communities in which the class had lived, worked, and traveled.

Ideas for Use

- "Let's Discuss" is useful for new or controversial topics.
- Using PowerPoint allows you to scan in portions of text or questions to spur classroom discussion.
- "**Let's Discuss**" sets the stage for classroom participation, so other group or active learning strategies may be used.
- This strategy may be used following another icebreaker to continue to build group process.

- I've used this strategy to summarize a section of study before going on to other topics. **Let's Discuss** opens the floor to questions, comments, and free interchange about the topic or material.
- **Let's Discuss** may be used as a segue to other topics, for review after breaks, or to reinforce key points. You can use it in the middle of a class when you sense the need for a break or some confusion on the part of the students.
- **Let's Discuss** may be the perfect strategy to use when you sense students puzzling over a **Muddiest Part.**
- This strategy changes the mood of a class from lecture to discussion. Simply saying "**Let's Discuss** . . . " gives the students license to participate.
- In academic settings, this strategy reinforces test materials, parts of the text to be reviewed, and areas that may be confusing. It helps students realize that they aren't the only ones having difficulty with a tough section.
- In nonacademic settings, **Let's Discuss** allows participants to share their experiences while learning from the experiences of others.

Self-test: How Creative Are You?

General Description   This strategy is most effective when students arrive at different times—for example, when some are unavoidably late and the rest of the class has already arrived, or when there is a prolonged or staggered registration period. **Self-test** also helps when the speaker is not quite ready. In this method, a quiz is distributed to the class. The quiz usually doesn't relate to the topic; it's meant to get creative juices flowing. I first encountered **Self-test** at a scout leader orientation, where it was used to break the ice and demonstrate the flexible and inquisitive mind needed to work with young boys.

Preparation and Equipment   You can copy the quiz out of this text. You can also scan it into PowerPoint or put it on an overhead projector, but students take it more seriously when they are working from their own copy.

Example of the Strategy at Work   Here is the quiz; the answers follow.

Creativity Quiz

1. A friend gives you two U.S. coins that equal 55 cents. One of them is not a nickel. What is the other coin?
2. How many species did Moses take on the ark?
3. Some months have 30 days, some 31. How many have 28?

4. How much dirt is contained in a hole 2 ft by 2 ft by I ft?
5. A farmer had 17 sheep. All but nine died. How many does he have left?
6. Each country has its own Independence Day. Do they have the 4th of July in England?
7. Is it legal in California for a man to marry his widow's sister?
8. How far can a dog run into the forest?
9. Two women are playing chess. They played five games and each won an equal number of games. There were no ties. How can this be?
10. An archeologist found two coins inscribed "46 BC." How old are they now?
11. How many Fs in this sentence: Fine infants' and children's shoes are the result of decades of scientific research combined with years of experience.
12. A patient has been injured in an automobile accident in which the patient's father was killed. The doctor refuses to operate because the patient is the doctor's son. How can this be?

ANSWERS

1. A nickel.
2. Moses wasn't on the Ark; Noah was.
3. All 12 months have 28 days.
4. None, it's a hole.
5. Nine.
6. There is a 4th of July is in every country.
7. No, he's dead.
8. Halfway, then he's running out of the forest.
9. They are not playing each other.
10. They are bogus, nothing is dated "BC."
11. Six lower and upper case or one upper case F.
12. The doctor is the mother.

Ideas for Use

- **Self-test** can be used any time your goal is not only to break the ice, but also to stimulate creativity, inquisitiveness, and a team spirit. It has been used in many teaching venues to open a discussion about creativity. Creativity is presented as a habit to be learned and cultivated, rather than as an innate or inherited trait.

- To hone test-taking skills, students may take this quiz and then discuss the need to read questions carefully. Invariably, some don't catch Moses versus Noah or some of the other subtle, but generally easy, questions.
- Froman and Owen[2] used a similar quiz in teaching about innovative methods to teach research. Their quiz, entitled "Logico-perceptual Thinking—A Test for Intelligence," was used as an assessment of validity. The authors administered several creativity questions and then discussed whether the results should be used to determine performance evaluations, pay raises, and other rewards. Subsequent discussions focused on the valid use of the quiz results in those situations, and on the valid use of tools to measure parameters outside their intended scope. The same quiz has been used to stimulate interest in research.
- You can do **Self-test** in pairs or trios as a way to build team spirit for future exercises.
- When flexibility is discussed, this quiz helps to drive home points such as "You need to be able to think differently." It's valuable in classes about conflict resolution, problem-solving, or nursing decision-making.
- A colleague* used the strategy to get the group started in a publishing workshop. She presented publishing as a process that requires flexibility and creativity, and asked the class to reframe the task and think about it a little differently. She then gave the following quiz, which the class worked on in pairs or trios. As a result, the students got to know one another and learned to regard publishing as a less formidable task.

1. How do you get a giraffe in the refrigerator?
   You open the door, put the giraffe inside, and close the door.
2. How do you get an elephant in the refrigerator?
   You open the door, take out the giraffe, put in the elephant, and close the door.
3. The Lion King has a party. All the animals come except one. Which animal doesn't go to the Lion King's party?
   The elephant—he's in the refrigerator.
4. A river is known to be full of crocodiles. You need to get to the other side. How do you get across?
   You wade or swim—all the crocodiles are at the Lion King's party.

---

*This exercise was originally conceived by Dr. Lucille Gambardella.

Using Toys, Prizes, and Props

General Description   This strategy is based on the premise that we learn with toys across our life span. Any physical object that creates a memory can assist with learning. These include props, visual cues, prizes, and objects that must be manipulated.

Preparation and Equipment   This strategy takes more preplanning than preparation. If you use props, toys, or prizes, they should have a relevant connection to the material. Ensure that the objects provide a visual cue for the class, to be remembered later. If you plan to distribute prizes or props to the entire class, select items that don't cost much, and make sure that you have enough for the entire class. If you use props, make sure they're large enough to be seen by the whole class.

Example of the Strategy at Work   **Toys, Prizes, and Props** have many uses. While teaching a class on stress management, I distributed Chinese finger traps from a discount toy store. Each student placed the index finger of each hand into one end of the trap. Then I asked the students to get their fingers out on their own. The students learned that the harder they pulled, the greater the tension on their fingers and the tighter the trap became. If they relaxed and allowed the trap to loosen, it slipped easily off their fingers. Many lessons may be taken from this exercise: The harder we try to deal with stress, the more stress we experience. The more we relax, the easier it is to deal with life's conflicts. And so forth.

Ideas for Use

- Use a sneaker to describe the learning process. In this exercise, students learn to tie their shoes all over again. First they are given a written description of how to tie a shoe and asked to forget that they know how to do it. They must use only the written guidelines. Then they are shown step-by-step pictures of shoe tying and asked to complete the job. Next, they are given a demonstration of shoe tying.

  Finally, the students learn the children's method: "Make one loop—that's the tree. Make another loop—that's the bunny. The bunny runs around the tree. Now he jumps in a hole under the tree. Now he comes out the other side and quickly runs away." We then discuss how slip-on shoes and Velcro™ fastenings have removed the challenges sneakers used to present and have created new ones.

  All of these examples provide visual cues about the learning process. They also provide nurses, nursing students, and clients with specific strategies for teaching and learning psychomotor skills.

- I've used a tool box to teach decision-making in nursing. Each tool represents a step in the process. In one demonstration, a hammer stood for psychomotor skills, the pliers for critical thinking, the screwdriver for a knowledge base, and the wrench for organizational skills. We then discussed the vital function of each "tool" and the negative effect on nursing care if a single one is missing.

  You can also show the class how the nurse uses each tool to arrive at a decision. Different tools represent assessment, diagnosis and analysis, planning, implementation, and evaluation. Again, each tool, representing each step of the nursing process, is important, but no one tool is more important than the others. For some jobs, tools must be used in a specific order.

- Gross[3] uses a Koosh® Ball to demonstrate how necessity breeds creativity. This toy was invented by a grandfather who enjoyed playing with his grandchildren. His wife frequently scolded them all about playing ball in the house for fear something would be broken. The grandfather's response was to create a ball out of rubber bands. The ball became the Koosh Ball. Not only is it safe for in-house play, but its inventor has made millions of dollars. I've used the same story to illustrate concepts such as creative problem-solving and personal achievement. I also use it to introduce a subject that may require an open mind, such as a change in agency policy, a difficult topic, or a problem warranting creative solutions or a shift in thinking.

- Give out "learning favors," much like party favors, to help students remember both the class content and the association with the favor when they look at it. Fortune cookies, magic tricks, and other novelties may be aligned with class objectives and encourage later recollection of the material.

- Use a flashlight to describe the nursing process. Let's say you turn on the flashlight and it doesn't work. At that point you make assessments. You determine whether there are batteries in the flashlight, the bulb is intact, the batteries are in correctly, and the switch is working. You then analyze all the data to develop a diagnosis of the problem. On the basis of your data, you determine that the batteries are dead and you plan to get a new set. You decide that dead batteries are the priority diagnosis and set about intervening, in this case replacing the batteries.

  In the evaluation phase, you discover that the light still doesn't work. You revise the care plan, using the cyclical nature of nursing decision-making, and discover that you may have inserted the batteries incorrectly. You plan, then intervene by reinserting the batteries. In your evaluation, when the light shines, you determine that the nursing diagnosis was correct and the problem is resolved.

- Bring a funnel to class. Use the funnel to describe the information coming into a nurse's consciousness. The nurse must churn through all of this information to effectively meet client needs, establish priorities, develop organizational skills, or learn a new specialty.

- Bring stretchy body parts found in the toy aisles of stores to reinforce assessment skills. Students are asked to describe the object using technical assessment terms and to discuss methods of physical examination relative to the type of body part. For example, a finger can be used to assess capillary refill, a foot can be used to assess pedal pulses, or an eye for the red reflex and condition of the cornea and color of the sclera.

- Combine several teaching strategies by using **Gaming** in class and providing prizes. Inexpensive trinkets, food products, nursing-related company giveaways, and tokens may be used. One summer, my children spent lots of good times "winning" boardwalk prizes for my students' fall games. Discount stores, toy stores, and magic stores can supply **Toys, Prizes, and Props.** Some mail-order companies gear their products specifically toward this type of market, in which large volumes of inexpensive items may be purchased.

- Bring a blender to class. I've used a blender to demonstrate the analytical part of the nursing process, in which all sorts of data must be mixed together to create a homogenized product, the nursing diagnosis. The blender can also denote the brain's role in neurological functioning, the need to mix different types of people in groups, and many other topics. This example illustrates the use of common household items to provide a visual cue.

- Show health-care equipment and let the students pass it around the room. This visual cue helps students to learn and understand difficult new equipment.

- Candy, gum, sugar-free products, and healthy snacks may be used. Food is always a welcome diversion.

- In teaching about conflict management and assertiveness, one colleague brings an assorted collection of stuffed and plastic sharks to class. She describes each to the class, emphasizing the characteristics and methods of dealing with well-dressed sharks, sharks in sheep's clothing, big sharks, little sharks, sharks with no teeth, and man-eating sharks. She passes out the sharks to the class and asks participants how they would react to and manage such a shark in their personal work environment.

- Bring bubbles to class. Bubbles are a common birthday party and wedding favor and may be purchased inexpensively at party stores. You need to connect the bubbles with class objectives: enhanced ventilation, celebration of a newly learned skill, or a creative teaching method. Then have the students blow the bubbles to provide a memory cue. You can also ask students to come up with their own associations—as long as the bubbles stay linked to course objectives or content.

- You can use bells and whistles to "reel in" the class after spirited group activities. You also can distribute them as visual cues; for example, whistles are effective in replicating breathing exercises. The bell or whistle may also be an auditory cue that you are moving to the next topic or section.

Starting with Games, Puzzles, and Brain Teasers

General Description   When students come to class, they see a puzzle, game, or brain teaser on the overhead or PowerPoint screen (Boxes 2–2, 2–3). This strategy is especially valuable for large classes, when lots of discussion and participation may become unwieldy. It provides an activity for early arrivals or students who don't know one another. Instructors can also pass out puzzles or games to get the thinking started.

Preparation and Equipment   You just need to find the brain teasers and have them available for the class, whether in audiovisual form or on paper.

Example of the Strategy at Work   Boxes 2–2 and 2–3 show only two of many possible brain teasers.

Ideas for Use

- Obviously, the examples shown have been used for pharmacology calculations. It can be used, though, for any material that has complex concepts or a **Muddiest Part.**
- E-mail the questions or brain teasers out to the class. Ask the class to bring the answers to the next class. You can also ask the students to answer you orally. Give prizes in front of the class to the ones who answer correctly. You can combine this strategy with **Admit Ticket.**
- Send the **Brain Teasers** out in the confirmation letter or in the registration materials. Use them to stimulate interest in a topic and discuss the answers in class as an icebreaker.

Box 2–2.
Brain Teaser

To Start You Thinking

1. A client is to receive 500 mg of ampicillin. It is diluted in 75 mL of normal saline solution and is to run for 45 minutes. The drop factor is 15 gtt/mL. What is the rate of the IV?
(Answer: 25 gtt/min)

2. A client is to receive 0.5 mg of naloxone, available in a 400-mcg/mL solution. What is the dose?
(Answer: 1.25 mL)

3. A client is to receive 500 mg of phenytoin, available in a 75-mg/mL solution. How many milliliters should he receive?
(Answer: 6.6 mL)

Box 2–3.
Brain Teaser

To Keep You Thinking

A client is to receive lidocaine at a rate of 2 mg/min. A 250-mL bottle of D_5W contains 1 gm of lidocaine. The IV set is labeled "Microdrip." At what rate should the nurse set the IV?
$1000 \div 250 = 4$ mg/mL
2 mg $\div 4 \times 1 = 0.5$ mg/min
Answer: $60 \times 0.5 = 30$ gtt/min

- Post the **Brain Teaser** to the class or to the organization's Web page. Provide prizes for those who enter the class with the right answer.

- Post answers to the class Web site or on a common class bulletin board.

- Include a **Brain Teaser** used in class as an extra credit option on an examination. This rewards class attendance, punctuality, and memory for the answer.

- If you include really difficult, "stumping" **Brain Teasers,** current class topics may not seem so formidable.

- Critical thinking texts provide puzzles and **Brain Teasers** relevant to nursing that may be adapted for any class content.

Common and Different

General Description   This may be one of my favorite icebreakers. It's valuable for students who don't know each other. Students are asked to form pairs or trios. Remind them not to select people they already know. They talk within their groups for a short time, perhaps 5 minutes. In that time, they must come up with four similarities and four characteristics unique to each group member. Invariably, gender, occupation, marital status, and parenting experience are mentioned.

Coming up with those eight characteristics requires students to delve somewhat into each others' lives. The most rewarding aspect of this method is that the students who do this exercise together become bonded for the duration of the class. Thus, collegiality increases among students who have not previously worked together. Be aware, though, that some students won't participate in this (or any other) icebreaker. However, this one is less threatening and appears to engage students more intensely than other strategies.

Preparation and Equipment   One of the greatest assets of this strategy is how much reward it produces with little effort. The only preparation you need is memory; just remember to introduce the strategy at the beginning of class. You can also prepare a screen with instructions that stimulate action and cut down on your need to give directions.

Example of the Strategy at Work   Box 2–4 shows one version of the slide I use for this exercise.

Ideas for Use

- Use **Common and Different** for nursing clinical groups or orientation groups. It's effective in creating a team spirit, especially when small numbers of participants know each other and others may feel left out.
- This exercise may be done in pairs, trios, or larger groups.
- You can alter the number—it doesn't have to be four—to fit the class time frame and objectives.
- **Common and Different** may be

Box 2–4.
Common and Different

- Talk to your neighbor on the left.
- Find four things you have in common.
- Find four differences between you.

What's harder—finding common ground or finding differences? Now you know each other!

used to open meetings. Even people who have worked together may discover some eye-openers when they reach out to discover each other's common points and differences.

- You can stimulate discussion after the exercise by asking the group, "Which was harder, finding commonalities or finding differences?" The answers may provide insight into the group process and composition.

- **Common and Different** may also generate discussion about differences and similarities, transferring to cultural, professional, ethical, or controversial topics.

Using Greeting Cards, Cartoons, and Pictures

General Description   This approach has been readily embraced by nurse educators. If you use it, you must be always on the lookout for greeting cards, cartoons, pictures, appropriate jokes or stories, and other material to open the class with a smile. The Internet has opened up a whole new world of e-mail jokes and other material. You can also search through calendars, newspapers, and magazines. The material should be amusing, relevant to the class content, and culturally and politically correct for general classroom use.

Preparation and Equipment   Materials may be photocopied onto transparency film, replicated freehand, or scanned into PowerPoint files. This strategy requires you to consider the fair use of copyrighted materials. Although attorneys provide varying opinions in their counsel on fair use, most stipulate that such materials can be used for educational purposes if you follow certain guidelines. You may not sell admission to a class solely on the basis of another's creative work, and you may not sell a copy of any written document that contains copyrighted material unless you have written permission. This means that PowerPoint slides or handouts should not include copies of such material or scans of cards, photos, or cartoons. Credit should always be given when it's appropriate.

Example of the Strategy at Work   I have used this strategy as an opening tactic. When students see slides with comics, pictures, or jokes on the screen, they feel welcomed and a friendly tone is set for the class. Here is one I have used and it was met with lots of laughter!

A frog goes into a bank and approaches the teller. He can see from her nameplate that her name is Patricia Whack. "Miss Whack, I'd like to get a $30,000 loan to take a holiday." Patty looks at the frog in disbelief and asks his name. The frog says his name is Kermit Jagger, his dad is Mick Jagger, and that it's okay, he knows the bank manager. Patty explains that he will need to secure the loan with some collateral. The frog says, "Sure, I have this," and produces a tiny porcelain elephant, about an inch tall, bright pink, and perfectly formed. Very confused, Patty explains that she'll have to consult with the bank manager and disappears into a back office.

She finds the manager and says, "There's a frog called Kermit Jagger out there who claims to know you and wants to borrow $30,000, and he wants to use this as collateral." She holds up the tiny pink elephant. "I mean, what in the world is this?" The bank manager looks back at her and says, "It's a knickknack, Patty Whack. Give the frog a loan. His old man's a Rolling Stone!"

Ideas for Use

- You can show Greeting Cards, Cartoons, and Pictures in the middle of lecture content to break up sections of material or as a transition into the next topic.
- Personal photos may be used with some content. Photos of others should always have a record of consent to use them for educational purposes.
- Again, the use of these materials requires the utmost in educator discretion. The strategy is effective in stimulating interest, but should not insult students or make them uncomfortable. You must use care with jokes and cartoons that use colorful language or innuendo, and you must keep in mind the purpose of the strategy. Discretion must also be exercised with fair use parameters.
- Frequent use of pictures from clip art, the Web, and scanning provides visual cues for learners. When creating handouts for class, make sure that you delete all pictures. This is important for legal reasons and also to decrease the time it takes to download handouts from the Web.

Why Are You Here?

General Description   This strategy explains itself, you simply ask **"Why Are You Here?"** before the start of a class session. You're trying to determine the students' goals for the class and examine their internal versus their external motivations for participating. You then can use this information in proceeding with the class.

This strategy sets clear boundaries, ensuring that expectations are in line with planned teaching topics or content. You may be able to gear class objectives toward student needs, or provide creative teaching strategies for less-motivated students. By determining the motivation level, you can employ creative teaching strategies to enhance internal motivation.

Preparation and Equipment   No preparation is involved. All you have to do is remind yourself to ask the question at the beginning of class.

Example of the Strategy at Work   I frequently use this strategy to open a semester or class. I show the sentence **Why Are You Here?** and solicit group responses (Box 2–5). The answers are sometimes amusing—for example, "Because my manager told me to come," "Because I have to," or "It's required." We then discuss what people want to learn from the class, how they want to be different at the end of it, or why they need the class to improve their current or future job performance. Some students have a sincere desire to be there and will answer, "Because nurses need to know this," or "I need to know this to go on in my career."

By collecting student responses, I am more able to assess the needs and abilities of the group. I then introduce class topics, class objectives, or both. This information allows all of us to determine whether the class will meet the students' needs and gives me the opportunity to change gears or clarify class objectives. It also reinforces what the class will include after a discussion of **Why Are You Here?**

Ideas for Use

- Use a flipchart to write down student responses. Go back to the flipchart at the end of class to determine whether most of the topics were addressed. You may want to briefly address topics that were missed.
- Some classes—for example, "the mandatories"—suffer from low levels of student motivation. **Why Are You Here?** gives you an opportunity to spur interest by using creative strategies, instilling motivation through stories and exercises, and discussing the reasons these courses are required.
- This strategy is effective in opening up classroom dialogue and getting students primed for later class participation.
- You can answer the question yourself, disclosing your love of teaching, your belief in the importance of the material, and your personal motivation to provide high-quality instruction.

> **Box 2–5.**
> ## Why Are You Here?
>
> - My boss told me to come.
> - What choice did I have?
> - A good nurse needs to know this.
> - I'm trying to get to the next step in my career.

Critical Thinking Exercises

General Description   **Critical Thinking Exercises (CTE)** are a great way to get the thinking juices flowing. Used early in the class, they encourage participation and ground the students in the class content. You can base them on class material or include them in the syllabus or in preparatory reading. This method encourages students to learn something about the topic before class, peruse the readings, and think about content before the class begins.

One frustration that students and novice nurses often encounter is the difficulty of setting priorities and "thinking like a nurse." Use of CTEs that pinpoint these priorities allows participants to determine what is integral to a problem. **Critical Thinking Exercises** in every class allow students to routinely practice internalizing and applying new concepts. This strategy is based on the THINK model crafted by Scheffer and Rubenfeld.[4] The model identifies the following components of the critical thinking process:

T: Total recall and memory
H: Habits of learning and thinking
I: Inquiry and in-depth thinking
N: New ideas and creativity
K: Knowing how one thinks and reflecting

Use of **Critical Thinking Exercises** allows students to use this THINK framework by:

- Recalling information
- Getting in the critical thinking habit
- Spending preclass time thinking about content
- Putting a new twist on known concepts
- Reflecting on content after class

Students also are able to assess their own learning before the rude awakening of an examination.

Preparation and Equipment   **Critical Thinking Exercises** can be introduced spontaneously or planned in advance. Questions such as "What role does the nurse have in caring for this client?," "What is the highest priority for the nurse and client?," and "How would the nurse cope with this situation?" allow students to see the "realness" of content and begin problem-solving.

Example of the Strategy at Work   For each nursing class, I provide four to six CTEs (Box 2–6). I make sure that these exercises, whether used to introduce or reinforce a topic, are well represented in the class

Box 2–6.
Critical Thinking Exercises

- A client receives a new diagnosis of diabetes mellitus (DM). The client doesn't need much insulin at this point. Why not?
- A client tells you her blood glucose levels are always within normal limits. She also tells you she only takes her insulin every other day to save money. What can you do to determine her past blood glucose values?
- Why are some organs more prone than others to hyperglycemic changes?
- What societal trends have influenced the increase in DM in the United States? What is the role of nursing in this issue?

objectives and on the evaluation material. I also make sure that my CTEs relate to test questions for academic classes. For continuing education classes, CTEs presented at the beginning of class help the students gain interest and give them a taste of the topics to be discussed.

Ideas for Use

- You may want to use this strategy at both the beginning and the end of class so you can evaluate learning and provide closure.
- I use the term **Critical Thinking Exercises or CTEs.** You may want to come up with another term, such as *Medical–Surgical Thinking Exercises,* to add interest and individuality for specific courses.
- These exercises may be adapted for e-mail use. You can make them sound friendly by calling them **E-mail Exercises.**
- **Critical Thinking Exercises** encourage attendance at class, especially when the topics lead to test questions. They also provide students with ready cues to use as study guides.
- Sometimes questions posed as **Critical Thinking Exercises** may be more user-friendly than objectives, which students may find formidable.
- For continuing education programs, include **Critical Thinking Exercises** in class brochures, registration letters, or class advertisements and brochures. Well-articulated CTEs entice students!
- In an academic setting, you may want to design **Critical Thinking Exercises** after examination questions, base examination questions on CTEs, or both. Either way, examination

questions and CTEs should reflect key concepts and learning priorities.

- These representative examples may be used as both **Critical Thinking Exercises** and examination questions:
  - How do hospitals make up the costs on an extended admission when diagnosis-related groups (DRGs) are in effect?
  - You make a medication error as a nursing student. Who is accountable?
  - Why does helping a client sit up ease respirations?
  - How do the signs of end organ perfusion differ in hypovolemic shock and in septic shock?
  - How can you assess the mental status changes in a client with hepatic encephalopathy?
  - What are the classic signs of hypoglycemia? Compare them with the classic signs of hyperglycemia.
  - A client is in congestive heart failure. What medications or classes of medications would you anticipate to be part of his care?
  - How do you assess pain in a nonverbal client?

Dress-up or Skits

General Description   At the beginning of class, the instructor dresses up or organizes a skit to provide relevant content or to introduce the class. These costumes or skits may be simple or elaborate and are focused on class objectives.

Preparation and Equipment   This strategy takes a lot of self-esteem and some preparation. Keep class objectives in mind so the costumes or props will enhance learning and retention. You can find dress-up materials by shopping in costume and thrift stores and by raiding the closets of your friends and family.

Example of the Strategy at Work   I have steered toward the simpler aspects of this strategy. I've worn some unlikely articles to help a class loosen up and focus on topics: a clown nose for a discussion of how humor is addressed in nursing theories; a boardwalk T-shirt with an anti-stress message for a class on nursing and stress; and a jester's hat to introduce nursing communication principles.

One group of students designed a class fundraiser with a sweatshirt showing "nursing diagnoses" (Fig. 2–2). I wore the sweatshirt to class and showed it as a slide to introduce the class to nursing diagnosis and analysis. Beginning nursing students have trouble embracing this rather dry concept, but the sweatshirt made it seem real and useful to their nursing

READ MY SHIRT:

Alteration in Mental Status
related to nursing school aeb…

- Weight Gain X 30 LBS.
- Increased Dementia
- Alternating constipation
  with diarrhea
- Sleep deprivation,
  2h q night x 10 weeks
- Social isolation
- Junk food dependency
- Instructor phobia
- Stooped posture
  (heavy book syndrome)
- Empty pocket syndrome

Problem?   Etiology?   Ident. Char.?

Fig. 2–2.   Read my shirt: Alteration in mental status related to nursing school.

careers. The strategy worked especially well because more senior students in the program had designed the shirt!

Ideas for Use

- A colleague arrived in class dressed in camouflage to represent the immune function of the T-cells and their responses to immunosuppression. This same faculty member used a superhero theme for the graduation address, wearing a belt, helmet, and other insignia borrowed from her preschool son to depict a "Supernurse."
- A well-known nursing speaker has been known to arrive at classes dressed as Mother Goose, a good fairy, and a nurse from ages past. Dressing up as part of the class theme truly does break the ice, but it also enhances retention of the material.

- Amusing hats, perioperative garb, historical costumes, scrubs, old uniforms, or any other odd clothing relaxes participants and helps you to teach serious material whimsically.

- Again, **Dress-up or Skits** can be as elaborate or as simple as you choose. The idea is to provide a visual reminder of the material—an image that novice nurses, students, or even experienced nurses can summon up to remind them of a topic.

- In addition to costumes and props, a script or skit helps with retention. Students can simulate a client interview or assessment, conduct a dialogue with a nurse from the past, respond to a mock resuscitation code, or act out the symptoms of a condition. I had two students videotape their skit of a client suffering from gastroesophageal reflux disease, demonstrating the signs, symptoms, and lifestyle issues that exacerbate the condition. We showed this video before class to reinforce the material for the session. Skits may be part of class assignments, extra credit, or performed on a volunteer basis, depending on the size of the class, the rapport among the students, and the time available.

Tell 'Em Once, Tell 'Em Twice, Tell 'Em Again!

General Description   Each class session should begin with an introduction and end with a summary. This teaching strategy is a great ice breaker. Repetition, a valuable teaching tool, allows students to organize their thoughts in a structured format and to hear the key priorities of the class again and again.

Preparation and Equipment   No special equipment is required. You should prepare a succinct, articulate introduction and summary to keep the students as focused as possible.

Example of the Strategy at Work   For each class I teach, I first introduce and later summarize the talk. When using PowerPoint, I create a screen for both the introduction and the summary (Boxes 2–7 and 2–8).

Box 2–7.
Drug Action: Introduction

- Why nurses need pharmacology
- Three phases of drug action
- Four pharmacokinetic processes
- Terms used in pharmacology
- Prototype medications
- Nursing implications of herbal therapy
- The nursing process
- Client teaching

Box 2–8.
Drug Action: Summary

- Determinants that affect drug therapy
- Nursing assessment and analysis
- Client teaching

Ideas for Use

- Use this method to begin and end every class. This gives your classes a level of predictability and closure.
- Many students live by the "get it, spit it, forget it" method of studying. Providing repetition of material improves long-term retention.
- Be warned that when students see the summary screen, they start packing up and leaving. I've started to put testing information, important learning hints, and other announcements on the last screen to discourage this behavior.
- Repetition is a sound principle of adult learning. **Tell 'Em Once, Tell 'Em Twice, Tell 'Em Again!** uses that principle as a framework for every class. It allows you to ensure that all content is being covered and that each area is reinforced.

Set the Stage

General Description   In the first few minutes of a class, whether in an academic or a clinical setting, the instructor primes the students for learning. **Set the Stage** is an ice-breaking strategy that establishes the ground rules, introduces the class, and sets the tone. This also is a great time for "housekeeping" details, setting important dates, and making necessary announcements. One colleague lamented that a student entered class with the question "Are you going to say anything important today?" **Set the Stage** lets the instructor ensure that something important will be covered in class!

In **Set the Stage**, the instructor may read poems or short stories, play music, discuss class policies, or introduce speakers. Many speakers prefer to introduce themselves; some let others introduce them. My personal preference is to avoid the common litany of educational and employment histories and ask speakers to decide what they'd like the class to know about them.

Preparation and Equipment   The equipment depends on the type of stage-setting method used. If you're reading a piece, you just need to bring it to class. If you're playing music, you need to prepare the cassette or CD player. You may copy a short excerpt of music to a CD to play for the class. An audio cable is needed with PowerPoint, or speakers can be attached to a laptop computer for large classes. When you copy short clips it's important to remember the rule of fair use, give credit to the composer and musicians, and contact your legal counsel with any questions.

Example of the Strategy at Work   I use one of my favorite stage-setting examples in a continuing education and academic class on adolescent health. At the beginning of this class, I read the following quotation to illustrate the characteristics of adolescent thinking. I adapted a story by Steinberg[5] and used it in an article I wrote on the "teen brain." This illustration, based on teen thinking, depicts some of the realities of treating adolescent clients:

You work with children with diabetes. You notice Caitlin is hospitalized—again! Caitlin is a 14-year-old with type 1 diabetes. This is her third admission in the last year—it is always the same. Caitlin gets busy with school and activities. She forgets to check her blood sugars. She doesn't know when her levels are high and when to check ketones. She forgets to calculate her carbohydrate-to-insulin ratio, doesn't correct her lows using her correction formula, and sometimes forgets her insulin altogether. She proceeds to be admitted with diabetic ketoacidosis. You sigh as you enter Caitlin's room. As you stand at her bedside you ask, "Caitlin, what were you thinking?" With wisdom far beyond her years or her recent behavior, Caitlin replies, "That's just it—I wasn't thinking!"[6] This confirms what you have believed all along—teens think differently!

Ideas for Use

- Play a popular song to set the tone for the class. You might use "Haven't Got Time for the Pain" by Carly Simon for a class in pain management, songs about heat for fever management, "Hope you Dance" by Lee Ann Womack for launching into publishing, and "These Are the Good Old Days" by Carly Simon to open a talk on the history of nursing. Some connections aren't as clear as others. For example, "Hope You Dance" embraces an active involvement in life and love. A colleague used this song to invite class participants to collaborate in publishing and enjoy the experience of writing for publication. Come up with your own tunes and play short excerpts to open the class. Song clips are especially effective in opening topics with an affective component.
- You can use a strategy called **Quiz About Me.** Tell the students several facts about yourself—years spent in nursing, your nursing specialty, your hobbies, or the way you spend your free time. Then turn around and ask them to tell the class the same facts about themselves. After a few students have shared their thoughts, ask, "How many people spend their time _____ ?" or

"How many people enjoy _____ ?," using the students' ideas to get to know the group. This strategy allows you and the class to get acquainted and puts you on a more human plane. It can take as little as 3 minutes.

- A colleague discusses using a "Stump the Professors" strategy to **set the stage**. Students are encouraged to come up with a fact or question to challenge the instructor. Keeping this strategy good-natured reinforces mutual respect and learning.
- **Set the Stage** is especially valuable in continuing education or staff development classes.
- Several ground rules in any class are important. In this day of cell phones, pagers, and direct-call phones, you need to send out a clear message about turning them off or silencing them. Even in the vibrate mode, the phone can be a disruption.
- Latecomers may also disrupt a class. Some instructors follow the theater model, in which the door is locked after the class has started. That way, students can't come in later and disturb the class. Of course, sometimes we're so glad to see students come to class, we may overlook infractions of punctuality.
- It's important to make clear that you and any speakers who come to class need quiet so they can present the material. All instructors have experienced the hassle of undercurrent conversations, which are very distracting for teachers and students alike. **Setting the Stage** for a professional class atmosphere can go a long way toward creating a fertile learning environment.

Setting Priorities

General Description   Setting priorities is one of the foremost challenges of nursing and nursing education. The more students learn, the more often they encounter this challenge. This strategy allows students to draw on their own experience, helps them clarify values, and validates the importance of thoughtful priority setting.

Preparation and Equipment   To use this strategy most effectively, give each student three index cards. If those aren't available, ask each students to tear off three small pieces of paper. You may want to prepare a PowerPoint slide to introduce the exercises.

Example of the Strategy at Work   I use this icebreaker to introduce a class on the planning stage of the nursing process. Each student is given three index cards. The class members list something that matters greatly to them, something they value highly, and something they believe is important—one item on each card. I ask the students to look at these three cards and arrange them in order of personal importance.

I ask the students to take their time to consider the criteria they use in priority ranking. Then comes the clincher: I ask them to rip up one card and throw it away. How does it feel to lose that thing they value so much?

The next step is to rip up another card. By now the whole class is groaning and suffering a sense of loss. We then discuss how it feels to lose things that we value. This topic leads us to the importance of setting priorities carefully, and in turn, how priorities depend on the individual. If there's time, students may share their real priorities, their reactions to loss, and the insight they gained from this exercise.

Ideas for Use

- **Setting Priorities,** like **Common and Different,** allows students to get to know each other.
- Students can share their thoughts with a partner, adding to the team-building quality of this exercise.
- This strategy demonstrates the difficulties of setting priorities in any situation that requires it.
- **Setting Priorities** demands a level a self-reflection and thought— students are asked to consider the impact of lifestyle or situational changes.
- To set client nursing priorities, list three to four client needs and have the students write them on cards. Then, as previously described, have students rip up cards and essentially develop a list of priorities among the concepts. This is a great way to introduce priority setting to novice students and nurses.
- In giving up what they treasure most, students may better understand the sacrifices imposed by aging, poverty, injury, or illness.
- For less aware students, this exercise provides a chance to practice both priority setting and the need to deal with loss.

Past Experiences with . . .

General Description   Some of the common reasons nurses enter the field are some past experience with health care, illness, or trauma; and acquaintance with nurses. Individual experiences can be valuable if shared among the group. This strategy simply calls for a brief discussion of the students' past experiences with any aspect of the class content.

Preparation and Equipment   No equipment is necessary. You just need to plan which topics to address and when to ask the questions during those classes.

Example of the Strategy at Work   **Past Experiences** works especially well with a group of 30 or fewer participants. I simply ask, "What have your past experiences with nursing been like?" or, "What past experiences have you had with nursing?" Surprisingly, students share very candid stories of both positive and negative experiences with nurses. Often these experiences, whether positive or negative, spark an interest in pursuing a nursing career.

Ideas for Use

- Seasoned nurses and continuing education students may be asked, "What past experiences have you had with nursing students?" as a way to generate discussion about the next generation of nurses.

- Personal experiences with illness, trauma, health care, and disability may provide a unique opportunity to share and learn. Although **Past Experiences** is introduced here as an icebreaker, students who know each other well may feel especially free to share intimate personal details.

- Sharing in a large classroom may be difficult. You can ask larger classes to reflect quietly on **Past Experiences** or to write down a short synopsis of their thoughts.

- Students in clinical groups may discuss hospital routines, nursing staff, and other subjects to generate discussion and share clinical experiences.

- For specific class material, it's effective to link the class topic with the students' past experiences. For example, if you're teaching a class on diabetes, you could ask, "What is your previous experience with diabetes?" or, "When you hear the word 'diabetes,' what do you think of?" This tactic introduces class material, provides a brief assessment of the class, and sets the stage for learning.

Be Prepared

General Description   Much as the Boy Scout phrase implies, students need to **Be Prepared** for class and learning. Often, though, they don't know how to prepare effectively for a class or learning session. Lack of preparation slows learning and frustrates the instructor and the class alike.

This strategy opens the class with a discussion of how students should **Be Prepared** for that particular session. You should share your hopes and expectations. The end of the class will include your suggestions on how the students should prepare for the next class. You'll use that closing strategy as the introduction to the next class.

Preparation and Equipment   An important element of **Be Prepared** is a critical analysis of what class preparation requires. Frequently we burden students with entire chapters and other long passages. Students may learn from experience that reading an entire assignment is a waste of time. Some will postpone the readings until after class so they can focus on information they've just heard. Meanwhile the instructor assumes that the group is prepared, only to be asked to spell some of the simpler words in the assignment.

Look over the course content and objectives and consider what preparation is essential for classroom learning. Abbreviated sections of readings; charts, pictures, or boxes; and questions and exercises within chapters often highlight key points of the content.

Example of the Strategy at Work   Nothing is more discouraging for an instructor than a class in which students walk in and ask, "What are we talking about today?" Obviously these students didn't do their readings or think about class objectives. When this happens, I use **Be Prepared** to help students get ready for subsequent classes.

At the end of one class and the beginning of the next, I focus on three to four aspects of each chapter or exercise that will assist in class preparation. For example, when presenting congestive heart failure (CHF) and medications, I ask students to review their pathophysiology notes about CHF. I remind them of the importance of the terms *preload, afterload,* and *contractility*. Then I tell them we'll be using these terms to describe the actions of selected medications. This technique sparks interest—now they understand the need to remember these words. I do this exercise a few minutes before class ends to keep the students from putting away their notebooks in the middle of my discussion.

Ideas for Use

- Textbooks are great resources for questions, terms to define, case studies, and chapter synopses.
- Sometimes just reading the chapter summary helps students get a glimmer of what the next class will cover. You should reinforce the importance of reading more deeply, but busy students may benefit from some shortcuts.
- Preparation is difficult to expect from busy nurses attending continuing or in-service education. Signs or e-mail messages hinting at discussion topics may spark interest in attending a class. The mention of words or concepts learned in nursing school and perhaps forgotten can also generate interest. This also is true if the content represents a new skill set or job expectation.
- Articles or outlines for class preparation may be posted online or in public areas. Some schools and agencies have found the rest rooms a great forum for educational materials! One academic setting calls this "Elimination Illumination."
- Gather some "Do you know?" questions under the **Be Prepared** heading. Post them on a sign or in an e-mail. They'll stimulate

questions, encourage thought, and increase the likelihood that your students will be prepared.

- Any material used to entice your students must be discussed in class and included in tests. This kind of follow-up is necessary to drive home the value of the strategy.

My Biggest Challenge

General Description   Students and practicing nurses may enter class in a passive mode, expecting the instructor to do all the work. **My Biggest Challenge** is a great way to "get the thinking machine" going and encourage participation in the active teaching strategies that follow. As in several other icebreakers, participants are asked to consider their biggest challenge—in life, nursing, school, or any other area. Tying this challenge into the class content reinforces that content and engages the students in active thinking about the material.

Preparation and Equipment   Little equipment is needed for this strategy. The only preparation is to plan when and how you'll ask, "What was your biggest challenge?" Your approach may vary depending on the size of the class.

Example of the Strategy at Work   I use this strategy to develop empathic skills about some of the challenges faced by health-care clients and their families. It's especially effective in the class dealing with spinal cord injury. I start the class by saying,

"Okay, class. First, before we address our topic for today, I want you to consider what is the biggest challenge you have encountered in your life." After several minutes of discussion about personal health and life challenges, I ask, "What challenges confront the client sustaining a spinal cord injury?" The class readily mentions paralysis, potential need for a ventilator, loss of bowel and bladder activity, sexuality issues, and many other challenges these clients face. Some may note depression and other psychosocial issues.

Continued discussion of spinal cord injury management may highlight technological advances, medical treatments, and prevention of complications. The importance of high-quality nursing care in confronting and surmounting these challenges reinforces the key role of the nurse in caring for a client with spinal cord injury.

This 5- to 10-minute introduction engages students in considering the personal experience of clients with spinal cord injury and the need to see the individual rather than the medical diagnosis. A brief comparison of personal challenges with those of clients who are ill or injured provides a meaningful perspective for beginning practitioners.

Ideas for Use

- This strategy attaches value to the students' experiences. Too often, students are never asked to share their own experience, level of knowledge, or perspective. **My Biggest Challenge** communicates respect for background and experience and allows everyone to participate actively in the group.

- This strategy works well at a post-conference after clinical rotations. The small group encourages sharing. Personal experiences may be compared and contrasted with those encountered in a clinical setting.

- Clinical groups often need some ice breaking if the participants don't know one another. **My Biggest Challenge** promotes discussion, focuses on personal abilities to meet challenges, and provides insight into the strengths and weaknesses of each group member.

- **My Biggest Challenge** is valuable for novice nursing students and anyone who doesn't understand the obstacles imposed by illness or injury. It gives learners a frame of reference for contact with clients who have different needs and perspectives.

Discussion Starters

General Description   As the title indicates, this strategy gets the ball rolling. It's really a catch-all for the different tactics instructors use to generate discussion.

Individual teachers often establish particular phrases to signal to students that it's time to start class. When students hear, "What are we discussing in class today?" "How many of you have cared for clients with _____ ?" or "What do your readings say about this topic?," they know it's time to learn. **Discussion Starters** engage the participants, begin the class, and alleviate any discomfort associated with the material.

Preparation and Equipment   Planning and rehearsing your statement is all you need to do.

Example of the Strategy at Work   In teaching a large class, I found my standard "Let's get started" doesn't always command attention as well as I'd like. I selected a statement to open every class: "Thanks for coming to class. Today we're going to talk about _____ ." Before long I noticed that the students saw this **Discussion Starter** as a signal for class. Much like the bell in grammar school, it ended personal conversation; suddenly the pencils were poised to write. Interestingly, the participants glared at students who were still talking or entering the classroom late.

Ideas for Use

- Use **Discussion Starters** any time you need to get the class's attention. It only takes one or two to disrupt an entire class, regardless of size. **Discussion Starters** provide an established signal that it's time to learn.
- In a continuing education program with several sessions, a **Discussion Starter** can tie material together or provide a segue between different parts of the class.
- **Discussion Starters** may be used in smaller classes in which you seek active participation. The statement lets the class know when they can share and when you would like to manage the discussion.

Now that you've broken the ice and set the stage for learning, you can sail into teaching with many creative strategies at your command.

References

1. Dellinger, S: Communicating Beyond our Differences. Jade Ink, Tampa, FL, 1996.
2. Froman, RD, and Owen, SV: Teaching reliability and validity: Fun with classroom application. Journal of Continuing Education in Nursing 22:88–94, 1991.
3. Gross, R: Peak Learning: How to Create Your Own Lifelong Program for Personal Enlightenment and Professional Success. Putnam, New York, 1999.
4. Scheffer, BK, and Rubenfeld, MG: A consensus statement on critical thinking in nursing. Journal of Nursing Education 39(8):352–359, 2000.
5. Steinberg, L. Is decision making the right framework for research on adolescent risk taking? In Romer, D (ed): Reducing Adolescent Risk. Sage, Thousand Oaks, CA, 2002, pp 18–24.
6. Herrman, JW: The teen brain as a work in progress: Implications for pediatric nurses. Pediatric Nursing 31(2): 144–148, 2005.

Personal Journal Pages

Chapter 3

Strategies for Large Classrooms

"The mediocre teacher tells. The good teacher explains. The superior teacher demonstrates. The great teacher inspires." —W.A. Ward

Challenges

- Inevitably, large classes include students with diverse learning styles, expectations, and attention spans.
- Large classrooms may present space and noise issues that impede creative teaching strategies and group work.
- Room lighting and size may challenge the instructor's ability to relate to students and establish eye contact. Sometimes the instructor may even have trouble seeing all the students and may feel isolated from the class.
- Physical distance in the classroom may create a formal and impersonal learning environment, making it difficult to engage all the students.
- An instructor in a large class may find it difficult to recognize students, recall their names, and relate to them in general.
- Because large classes encourage anonymity, students may be unprepared, uninvolved, or inattentive.
- Conversely, students may find large classes frustrating because the instructor can't give personal attention or be aware of individual learning needs.
- Less assertive students may be reluctant to participate in large classes, leaving their questions unanswered and their contributions unshared.
- Students who don't know each other may be uncomfortable with, and therefore resistant to, creative teaching strategies.

In a large class, you need strategies to help you increase your students' comfort, engage them in the material, and stimulate their interest. If you intersperse the traditional large lecture class with quick, uncomplicated strategies, you will reinforce concepts, grab your students' attention, and create a warm and inviting learning atmosphere.

IDEAS

Short Clips

General Description   Showing short film clips in the middle of class is an attention-grabbing way to emphasize a point and break up material. Most students today watch television and frequent movie theatres, so this strategy capitalizes on their frame of reference. **Short Clips** may come from commercials, television serials about health care, or popular movies. Clips may portray positive or negative images of nursing and health care related to class topics, or depict patient responses to crisis or illness.

This method promotes thinking and direct application of information. For **Short Clips** to have the greatest effect, you should focus on class objectives and develop "thinking questions" or exercises to provide focus. See Herrman, "Using Film Clips to Enhance Nursing Education,"[1] for more details.

Preparation and Equipment   You can use various methods to present **Short Clips.** Cueing of VHS videos or DVDs allows you to play the clip in class, provided a VCR or DVD player is available. DVD software lets you bookmark selected clips and play them on a laptop or desktop computer. The newest version of PowerPoint lets you add cueing signals to presentations to trigger the appearance of specified scenes. Other software packages let you copy short clips onto a CD. Fair use may be interpreted to allow the making of limited, short clips, used during class, to meet learning objectives. This method requires a significant amount of technological knowledge. Check your agency resources for support in this area.[1]

Example of the Strategy at Work   I frequently use this strategy to teach both in the classroom and in staff development settings. Popular movies (see Table 5–1) provide fertile ground for discussion of health and illness issues, current societal conflicts, and day-to-day living.

Examples I have used include *Pearl Harbor, Patch Adams, A Beautiful Mind, Save the Last Dance, Remember the Titans, Young Frankenstein,* and others. I've used *John Q* to discuss access to health care and the use of medical jargon. *How the Grinch Stole Christmas* demonstrates the stages of change as the Grinch is transformed into a caring soul. I have used scenes from *A Beautiful Mind* to carry though the entire nursing process discussion, providing examples of assessment, analysis, planning, implementation, and evaluation. *Patch Adams* can demonstrate what not to do in nursing grand rounds, the value of humor in wellness, and the use of group therapy in the care of clients with mental health issues.

Prepare thinking questions in advance, show them to the students before you show the clip, and discuss them afterward. Appropriate questions include "What are the nursing implications of this clip?," "How should a nurse respond in this situation?," and "How does this clip relate to the subject matter of today's class?"

Ideas for Use

- Tired learners, both students and working nurses, may appreciate the use of film clips to enhance the discussion topic and provide entertainment.
- You can use **Short Clips** in each class or in just one. You can show several clips from one video in a single session and discuss related topics as the story unfolds.
- Make sure that you reinforce points of discussion, or "thinking questions," so that students see the film clips as a learning method, not just time off from class.
- **Clinical Decision-making Exercises** or **Critical Thinking Exercises,** discussed in other chapters, may be combined with this strategy.
- Movie clips can stimulate engaging conversations because videos and television are such a comfortable method of communication for today's learners.
- Some video clips depict clinical signs and symptoms that are difficult to demonstrate in the classroom. *A Beautiful Mind* contains a scene showing seizure activity; *Awakenings* demonstrates extrapyramidal, parkinsonian symptoms; and *Patch Adams* shows catatonic behavior.

Read a Story

General Description   This commonly used strategy allows the instructor to use some creativity by interjecting fiction, poetry, and other literature into class content. Information from popular books, business texts, parenting books, personal nursing stories, comics, newspaper columns, and children's literature provide great teaching fuel and add relevance to potentially dry content. Business success guides may offer inspirational and encouraging messages. Children's books may provide poignant stories about life conflicts, illness, death, or personal experiences from the eyes of a child—often very compelling for adult learners.

Preparation and Equipment   Stay alert, especially if you go into a bookstore or pass a newsstand. Resources providing interesting quotations or passages may appear at surprising moments.

Example of the Strategy at Work   The story in Box 3–1, given to me by a colleague, helps me when I discuss poverty and global health issues. I hope that you can also use it.

For another example of this strategy, I read from an 1885 nursing text-book that I found at an antique show. I have read many excerpts about nursing in that era, and we've discussed the significant advancements made since that time. Here is a selection I especially like when discussing nursing research:

Try to find out why things are done, to be familiar with the under-lying principles as well as details of practice. Learn to nurse by reason rather than by rule, for no rule can be laid down to which exceptions will not arise. Do not fancy that after you have been through a train-ing-school you will know all there is to know about nursing; in fact, you will only have been taught how to learn, how to appreciate and profit by experience which you will get. Every new case will teach you something new.[2]

Ideas for Use

- Don't rely exclusively on books. Newspaper articles, columns, and editorials also provide great material.
- Nursing journals have begun to publish works reflecting the art of nursing. Poetry, haiku, and short stories may carry powerful messages.

Box 3–1.
A Village of 100

Imagine the world reduced to 100 people. Fifty-one would be female. Seventy would be nonwhite. Eighty would live in substan-dard housing. Seventy would be unable to read. Fifty would suffer from malnutrition. One would be near death and one would have just been born. One would graduate from college and no one would have a computer. Fifty percent of the world's wealth would be in the hands of six people—all living in the United States.

- The coloring book *I Might Be a Nurse*[3] is a great resource for early nursing students.
- Children's books such as *The Fall of Freddy the Leaf*[4] and *Bob and Jack: A Boy and His Yak*[5] provide insights into children's concepts of aging and death. *The Three Little Pigs From the Wolf's Point of View*[6] shows how viewing problems from various perspectives can illuminate the real meaning of an issue.
- Old copies of *Cherry Ames* books and other novels about nurses may provide historical images of nursing. The Springer Publishing Company has republished four books of the *Cherry Ames* series in a boxed set with introductions by Harriet Forman.[6] Other books in this series are available from online retailers.
- Two Golden Books, *Nurse Nancy*[7] and *Doctor Dan,*[8] can assist students in delineating professional roles. Bond[9] discusses the use of *Nurse Nancy* in a professional nursing course as a means of teaching nursing knowledge and the nursing process.

Use the Star

General Description   Students have a difficult time determining priorities and identifying key study materials. Novice nursing students frequently highlight every word in the chapter and can't distinguish vital information from the rest.

In this easy strategy, stars are used to distinguish the most important material from the rest. Asking students to **Use the Star** will give them useful visual and auditory prompts. You can use stars in PowerPoint presentations or traditional handouts, or you can simply ask the class to "put a star next to this." Stars highlight important material to be used later as study tools.

Preparation and Equipment   No preparation is required. Stars may be added either before or during class.

Example of the Strategy at Work   This strategy can be used spontaneously. During class preparation, I've added PowerPoint stars to areas that need emphasis. I realized this strategy was a success when a teaching assistant told the class, "Pay attention to the stars."

It's important to make sure that test questions coincide with starred material; if you don't, students will learn not to trust the stars. This doesn't mean you need to "teach to the test"; however, **Use the Star** keeps the focus on key points and helps the students identify potential test questions (Fig. 3–1).

Ideas for Use

- **Use the Star** is a great way for faculty to ensure that tests represent key factors in class content. Often tests are constructed before

ETHICAL PRINCIPLES

- Beneficence
- Nonmaleficence
- Autonomy
- Paternalism
- Justice
- Allocation of resources
- Informed consent
- Accountability
- Confidentiality
- Self-determination
- Fidelity

Fig. 3–1.   Use the Star to illustrate important points in class.

the first class meeting, making it difficult to ensure that vital facts are tested. By basing your test questions on starred material, you can stick to the important facts, ensure test content validity, and avoid minutiae. You can also be sure that the students know what information matters the most.

- Ask your students what information deserves to be starred. Use frequent pauses as an opportunity to ask, "Okay, what facts covered in the last 20 minutes deserve a star?" Given this opening, students will revisit and repeat information while developing skills in priority setting.

- This strategy is important for new nurses or those new to a clinical specialty. Even nurses who have been practicing for a while may need to learn the priorities specific to an unfamiliar clinical area. Starred material provides a way for nurses at all levels to focus on new and vital information.

- **Use the Star** ensures that students are actively writing and attending to notes during class.

Case Studies: Quickie

General Description   The use of case studies in nursing education is well documented. Nurses and nursing students share and learn by clinical anecdotes, real-life experiences, and "war stories." Case studies teach reality-based information within a story developed according to specific class content and objectives.

The drama of a case study allows nurses and nursing students to embrace information on a human plane. Because the case study is fictitious, the teacher can mold it to include relevant details and emphasize key information.

Case studies may take a while to write but can be used over and over again. They can be as brief or extensive as class and preparation time allow. The next several strategies describe several uses of case studies in teaching. Case studies work well with large classes when other creative strategies prove unwieldy, but they may be used in any teaching venue. **Quickie Case Studies** are just that—a brief introduction to the client and the main clinical issue. **Quickie Case Studies** may be used to introduce topics, segue from one area to another, emphasize priorities, or to show how concepts fit together.

Preparation and Equipment   This strategy takes more cognitive effort than anything else. Once a lecture is written and the content and objectives are established, you can write your **Quickie Case Study.** This can be read out loud, written onto a slide, or included in a handout.

Example of the Strategy at Work   I use **Quickie Case Studies** to differentiate type 1 and type 2 diabetes mellitus. That way the class can differentiate the diagnosis, characteristics, and management of the two types. This **Quickie Case Study** provides a transition in the discussion from type 1 to type 2 diabetes, highlighting several of the differences and nursing implications.

Quickie Case Study

Type 1 Diabetes Mellitus

A.C., a 6-year-old boy, is taken to the pediatrician by his mother. He says he feels "bad" and "tired all the time." His mother notes that he has been drinking and eating a lot and is "always going to the bathroom." She adds that he appears thinner and lacks his usual energy. She also comments that his breath smells sweet. A peripheral blood glucose level is 450 mg/dL. A.C. is referred to the endocrinology clinic.

Quickie Case Study

Type 2 Diabetes Mellitus

J.C. is a 58-year-old man with a history of hypertension and cerebrovascular accident. He is African American and is 40 lb overweight. His mother is being treated for type 2 diabetes mellitus. J.C. has been drinking and urinating more than usual but says he feels well. He is on disability leave from work and lives a sedentary life. When asked about his diet, he replies, "I eat what I want to. I don't like to diet." Routine blood work reveals hyperglycemia, and he is referred to the endocrinology clinic.

Ideas for Use

- Use **Quickie Case Studies** to open or close a class session. They also can be used as a transition from one topic to another, ensuring students are caught up with the changes in class subjects.
- Use case study content to provide a test review. **Quickie Case Studies** can provide the context for later test questions.
- One hazard of using case studies is the possibility that the students will overgeneralize. It's important to emphasize that the case study is an example of issues and characteristics. Novice students or nurses may assume that all clients with certain characteristics encounter the same issues. Make sure you include a preliminary statement that the case represents a prototype rather than a "standard client" with all the same issues.
- **Quickie Case Studies** are valuable when clinical pictures are closely aligned or when differences are subtle. Students can analyze the differences within a short, tight framework.
- Handouts may include the case study and appropriate study questions. You can combine **Quickie Case Studies** with **E-mail Exercises** or **Online Discussions.**
- Case study strategies may be coupled with **Group Thought, Think-Pair-Share,** and **Teaching Trios**.

Case Studies: Preclass

General Description   **Preclass Case Studies** are especially valuable if some preliminary study is needed before class. Examples include technical information that may depend on background reading, preparation for class, or classes that need to cover more content than time allows. **Preclass Case Studies** also reinforce learning by requiring students to read, write, and hear the material.

Preparation and Equipment   **Preclass Case Studies** need to be written in advance and should be fairly detailed. These case studies then are posted on the Internet, included in the class workbook, or distributed as a handout. Class time is set aside to discuss the case study and the accompanying questions.

Example of the Strategy at Work   I developed this strategy while teaching a class on pediatric gastrointestinal problems. The class contained far more content than I could cover in 2 hours.

I decided to develop a cleft lip and palate case study. This study allowed an extensive discussion of the medical, surgical, nursing, and multidisciplinary approach to managing cleft lip and palate disorders. Students were instructed to read the case study before class and to underline key words associated with organic changes, assessments, and management and nursing considerations. Study questions, discussed in class, were based on the case study information.

Students who had prepared well understood the rather brief discussion that reflected the case study. Students who didn't prepare appeared lost, especially when I mentioned that the test questions on this content would be drawn directly from this case study. The next time I used a **Preclass Case Study** on another topic in that class, I found most of the students prepared, and we completed the material quickly.

Ideas for Use

- Use **Preclass Case Studies** when you need to spend less time on a single topic.
- **Preclass Case Studies** help when preparation before class is vital to understanding material. Have participants read the case study, answer key questions, and hand in the answers on admission to class (see **Admit Ticket**).
- **Preclass Case Studies** may be used in continuing education and staff development settings to ensure that all participants are "on the same page." If you include a case study in registration materials, students can look over the case, do background reading, and consider answer options.
- Ensure that the topic of a **Preclass Case Study** is represented on a test or examination. Use the basic elements of the case study to develop multiple-choice items or quiz questions.
- Case studies done before class may be part of an **E-mail Exercise** or an **Online Discussion.**

Case Studies: Interspersed

General Description   Like the previous case study formats, the **Interspersed Case Study** allows for a short pause in the lecture to discuss a case. These mini-cases are simply used to reinforce key points or to emphasize important content. They are based on single concepts and are directed toward "starting the thinking machine" about one area of discussion. You can design them to clarify difficult concepts or to help students establish priorities among conflicting demands.

Preparation and Equipment   Write the **Interspersed Case Study** after you've written the lecture and established the content and objectives. You can read the study out loud, write it onto a PowerPoint or any other type of slide, or include it in a handout.

Example of the Strategy at Work   I use the **Interspersed Case Study** to break up lecture content and to reinforce key information. In a class on stress management I found that students often internalized class content into their own personal situations; they rarely considered the role of the nurse in helping clients to cope with stress. The **Interspersed Case Study** asks students to consider what sort of assistance they can offer this client. They're called on to identify his major stressors, the signs and symptoms of stress, and potential nursing interventions to use in stress assessment and management. Using an **Interspersed Case Study** helps students begin to assimilate their role as practitioner.

Interspersed Case Study

A Stressed Client

K.L. is a 36-year-old man. He is married and has four children, 1 to 5 years old. He smokes two packs of cigarettes per day, is 20 lb overweight, does not exercise, and admits to drinking five or six alcoholic drinks every day. He expresses frustration with his job, family situation, and life in general. He feels that stress is his most significant problem.

Ideas for Use

- Use **Interspersed Case Studies** any time you believe students are finding information difficult or confusing. Put the information on a personal plane to help them understand complex concepts.
- Conclude a class with a brief **Interspersed Case Study** to reinforce information.

- To discuss the case study and related **Critical Thinking Exercises,** have students split into groups for **Think-Pair-Share, Teaching Trios,** or **Group Thought.**
- If using **Group Thought,** choose cases that differ slightly to help students understand the subtleties of different situations. Ask students to report back to the class with conclusions (see **Group Thought**).
- If you're using objective examinations, use **Interspersed Case Studies** in each class to emphasize test material. Help students see the entire spectrum of the nursing process by asking questions that represent each step. This strategy is important in preparation for the NCLEX®.

Case Studies: Continuing

General Description   **Continuing Case Studies** develop through-out the class as content is presented. I like to expand on the same case study throughout one class session. Doing this allows my students to get to know the client, and revisiting the study creates a holistic picture of the client and his or her nursing care. **Continuing Case Studies** provide a human element—the subject of the case study becomes an old friend to be revisited—and students can apply the information as it's discussed.

This strategy is especially valuable when single, complex topics are taught in one session. The case continues to develop as content becomes more complex, as the client's status changes, or as the information branches off into related topics. The **Continuing Case Study** is intro-duced at the beginning of class, discussed during class, and used to sum-marize issues at the end of the session. **Continuing Case Studies** are beneficial when the course of a complex condition is discussed, allow-ing students to witness the diagnosis, assessments, treatment, client response, and nursing implications.

Preparation and Equipment   Write the **Continuing Case Study** after you've written the lecture and established the content and objectives. Like **Interspersed Case Studies, Continuing Case Studies** can be read out loud, written onto any type of slide, or included in a handout. I like to decorate my slides with humorous drawings, which help students remember the material.

Example of the Strategy at Work   I have used **Continuing Case Studies** to teach concepts across the nursing process, such as pain assess-ment and management. In the first slide, I present the client.

Continuing Case Study

A Postsurgical Client

L.W. is 13 years old and has scoliosis. She had a posterior spinal fusion today. The surgery took 6 hours, and the incision is 18-in. long. She is on postoperative bedrest for 24 hours, has two IVs and a Foley catheter, and is receiving patient-controlled analgesia.

We then discuss pain assessment and the physiological, behavioral, and subjective criteria we use to measure pain. Then the client's assessment information is presented.

Continuing Case Study

Postsurgical Assessment

- Denies severe pain
- Pulse 130 bpm, respirations 36/min, blood pressure 118/88 mm Hg
- Restless, refuses to move, moans with turning and care
- Verbalizes pain at 7 on a scale of 1 to 10
- Refuses to breathe deeply or cough
- Reports pain at incision and graft sites
- Parents at bedside—very anxious

The lecture then turns to pain management. Pharmacological and nonpharmacological methods are discussed. I reinforce the lecture with a slide.

Continuing Case Study

Management

- Patient-controlled analgesia with continuous morphine
- Morphine bolus with care and position changes
- Distraction
- Dark, quiet room
- Warm cloth on forehead
- Client and parent education

Finally, I present the concept of evaluation as integral to pain assessment and management. In summary, we discuss the importance of evaluating and reevaluating pain from the client's perspective.

Continuing Case Study

Evaluation

- Verbalizes pain at 4 on a scale of 1 to 10
- Logrolls freely in bed; Foley catheter discontinued
- Using female urinal
- Breathing deeply and coughing
- Vital signs within normal limits
- Sipping liquids
- Interacting with parents
- Watching TV
- Expressing fears but excited about getting out of bed tomorrow

---

Ideas for Use

- **Continuing Case Studies** work well for single topics in which the content develops detail and complexity throughout the class. Extensive classroom time is often needed for topics such as shock, cardiac emergencies, the surgical process, and various aspects of cancer management.
- **Continuing Case Studies** may be used for examination review to reinforce material that may have been taught several weeks ago.
- This strategy is especially valuable in continuing education and staff development, in which experienced nurses learn best with real-life scenarios. Providing the case study with discussion points every 15 minutes or so appeals to listeners and accommodates the attention span of busy learners.
- Have students develop a **Continuing Case Study** as part of an **E-mail Exercise** or **Online Discussion.**

Case Studies: Unfolding

General Description   This innovative strategy was developed and documented by Glendon and Ulrich.[10] Their book contains more than 50 case studies. Each story divulges an increasing amount of details during the course of the study. As the plot thickens and the story unfolds, students are asked to consider the many facets of the client's care.

The merit of these cases lies in the lifelike, dynamic nature of the stories, which weave in clinical status changes and the results of assessments and interventions. As the case develops, the student must consider the increasingly complex details and use them to influence decisions. The class discusses the study as it grows more complex. Educators may use the published **Unfolding Case Studies,** which represent all nursing specialties, or create their own. Those included by Glendon and Ulrich represent all nursing specialties, various nursing settings, and different phases of clinical expertise.

Preparation and Equipment   As with other case studies, **Unfolding Case Studies** need to be developed as part of class preparation. After the class is organized, an **Unfolding Case Study** can be developed to include its various aspects.

Example of the Strategy at Work   I have used several of the cases developed by Glendon and Ulrich.[10] The book includes these cases and guidelines for using case studies. The one I especially love involves two nursing students and highlights the need for patient confidentiality.

I'll summarize the case: Two student nurses are working in labor and delivery. Each has a client. One mother discusses her husband Jim and his steadfast nature. The other mother talks about her boyfriend Jim and their future marriage. A man named Jim comes to visit both, and the nursing students decide he is the same man and spread rumors all over the unit. The visiting Jim turns out to be both women's pastor, and the students learn the lesson of jumping to conclusions and the hazards of breaching patient confidentiality.

Students love the drama associated with this case. They recognize the students in the study and compare it with their own professional role in the clinical area. I use **Think-Pair-Share** with this case to have students discuss the legal and ethical implications of this issue.

Ideas for Use

- Develop your own **Unfolding Case Studies** to emphasize key points. Add more information to the case as it unfolds to challenge students further and to reinforce important issues.
- Ask students critical thinking questions through **E-mail Exercises** or **Online Discussions** to keep them thinking.
- Use the **Unfolding Case Studies** developed by Glendon and Ulrich[10] to enhance your personal teaching materials.
- Use the unfolding nature of these cases to demonstrate unexpected yet common changes in client status. Discuss the postoperative

client who develops a wound infection, the client who develops congestive heart failure after a myocardial infarction, a client going through the stages of sickle cell crisis, or the laboring mother who experiences a placental abruption. By adding details as the case unfolds, you'll introduce students to the dynamic nature of client care and the need for ongoing assessments and decision-making.

Use the Book

General Description   This strategy encourages both students and instructors to **Use the Book.** Nursing education and other textbooks often include resources that go unused because of time, lack of knowledge, or just habit. In addition, students frequently use class notes to study for a test; today's learners don't seem to read to supplement knowledge.

Use the Book encourages use of the ancillary resources included with books. Many texts offer critical thinking exercises, test questions, CD-ROMs, and scenarios; publishers encourage authors to develop these because they make textbooks more marketable. Probably the greatest bene-fit of this strategy is that students learn the hidden uses of their textbook. Encouraged, they go back and **Use the Book** to learn material and study for the tests.

Preparation and Equipment   The only preparation for this strategy is to peruse the text and view the available resources. Use exercises that enhance class content or align with class objectives. This strategy may use key text-book information—boxes, charts, tables, examples, and pictures—which is then reinforced in class. By citing page numbers, scanning pictures into the lecture slides, using publisher-developed audiovisuals, and asking students to use the resources in the book, you emphasize the value of the book and its features.

Example of the Strategy at Work   This strategy can enhance learning in two ways. The first method simply uses the resources available to rein-force content. For pharmacology, I've used the case studies at the back of the chapter, and others, to summarize the class content. The case scenarios were geared toward lesson content and asked poignant questions related to the material.

Another way to use this strategy is to scan in pages of the book and selected information. I scanned in a box from the readings with the steps of case management. You may also ask the students to open their text-books to a page with the list of these steps. Then develop a case study using the information. The slides help students **Use the Book** and apply it to a case study you've developed. Following is an example in which I applied the steps of case management to a class-related study.

The Case Management Process

You are a nurse caring for C.C., a 14-year-old boy who sustained a spinal cord injury in a motor vehicle accident. He has a tracheostomy, is dependent on a ventilator, and is wheelchair bound. Use the steps of the case management process to consider his needs.

Ideas for Use

- Most textbooks provide a wealth of material that you can use to reinforce your teaching. Test questions, case scenarios, critical thinking exercises, and test banks may all be used to enhance classroom discussion.
- Students can use text resources in studying for tests and to clarify **Muddiest Parts.** Once they get comfortable with all the resources a book provides, students may become more eager to use it for class preparation and to do the assigned readings.
- Some students need the reinforcement of a postclass review. **Use the Book** gives them tangible exercises or review materials to look at after class. By reinforcing what they've learned in class, students can study in small, manageable chunks and avoid the last-minute cram before examinations.

Worksheets

General Description When we think back to our grammar school roots, some of us recall **Worksheets** as an important study tool, classroom activity, and teaching strategy. These valuable tools take some time to prepare in advance, but you can use them in class again and again.

Preparation and Equipment Class material must be prepared in advance so the **Worksheets** supplement the class content and increase the students' active participation in class. They also supplement student notes and PowerPoint handouts.

Example of the Strategy at Work Table 3–1 shows a worksheet I used for a discussion of pulmonary deficits with cystic fibrosis.

I've used this worksheet to clarify complex conditions such as the pulmonary deficits associated with cystic fibrosis. Other topics conducive to **Worksheets** include endocrine disorders, arterial blood gases, acid–base balance, and dysrhythmias. I try to leave off arrows indicating elevations or decreases in lab values or symptoms and to omit several words in each block of the **Worksheet.** When the students realize I'll be giving them the

Table 3–1 Management of Cystic Fibrosis: Pulmomary Changes

Pathophysiological Problems	Signs and Symptoms	Management and Nursing Implications
Short-Term Respiratory Changes		
_____ Mucus (viscosity, amount)	_____ Dyspnea	CPT, P&PD
		CBD, percussor vests
_____ Dilatation	_____ Cough	Exercise
_____ Fibrosis	_____ Aeration (especially lower lobes)	Forced fluids
_____ Ciliary action	_____ Wheezes	Adequate nutrition
_____ Mucus stasis	_____ Fatigue (hypoxia)	Bronchodilators
_____ CO_2, O_2 exchange	_____ Respiratory rate	Antibiotics (inhaled) Tobramycin
_____ Leukocyte-rich sputum	_____ Symptoms of URI	O_2 (low-liter flow)
_____ Risk for infection	_____ Sx of pneumonia	Expectorants, flutter valves
Long-Term Respiratory Changes		
_____ Fibrosis	_____ Sx of atelectasis	Relaxing
_____ Organ function	_____ FEV1	Forced exhalation (huffing)
_____ Potential for pneumothorax	_____ FCV	Nebulizers
_____ Cor pulmonale, pulmonary hypertension	_____ Barrel chest	Dornase alfa
_____ Multidrug resistance	_____ Clubbing	Ibuprofen (to decrease inflammation)
	_____ Signs of respiratory distress	Home care: Timing, skills, equipment
	_____ Rhonchi	Surgical management: lung transplant

CBD = coughing and deep breathing; CPT = chest physical therapy; P & PD = percussion and postural drainage; Sx = symptoms; URI = upper respiratory infection missing information, they listen more actively as they complete the **Worksheet** during class.

Another way to use a **Worksheet** in class is to combine this strategy with **Case Studies** and **Group Thought.** In this combined exercise, I provide the students with the following case and a copy of a blank incident report. Students fill in the components of the incident report and learn a valuable lesson about this part of professional nursing.

Medication Incident Report Case Study

You are a new nurse providing care to a client. The client's name is Jack Jones. His medical record number is MR6-798543, the date is 2/5/04, and the unit is 6 North at Smith Hospital. Your client is ordered to receive D5/0.45 normal saline solution by peripheral IV at 75 mL/h. A physician writes an order at 0645 to include 20 mEq of potassium chloride (KCl) in each 1000-mL bag of IV fluids. This order is not transcribed by the night shift nurse.

At 1600 in your chart review, you notice the order and realize that the client has not received the KCl. The physician is called. You draw a blood sample and find that the client's potassium level is 3.0 mEq/dL. The physician orders potassium added to the IV, and a potassium rider is hung.

Four hours later the serum potassium level is 3.9 mEq/dL. The client is asymptomatic and has suffered no long-term effects. The family is not notified, and documentation is limited to the lab results and the client's toleration of the added potassium.

Using the incident report sheet, complete the demographic information on the first page. Using the data in this case study and your personal experience, discuss the outcomes, parameters (contributing factors), and potential actions that could be taken in this case.

Ideas for Use

- To make this strategy work, you need to encourage active learning. **Worksheets** may be constructed from class lectures with blanks where some content should be. By prompting students, **Worksheets** require them to fill in the blanks, complete tasks, participate in class, and look up references and any needed information.
- **Worksheet** alternatives are "no-count quizzes," matching exercises, case studies with questions, and informational charts.

- Provide **Worksheets** in advance in syllabi, class workbooks, or on Internet-based classroom resources.
- Ask students to prepare by completing the **Worksheet** before class. Reward participation with prizes or recognition.
- Including a **Quickie Quiz** or a **Quiz that Counts** will reinforce both the material and the importance of preparation for class.
- This strategy can help you construct tests because it focuses on key information that must be revisited during the course.
- For continuing education, **Worksheets** may accompany registration materials. Participants can prepare for the class, think about its content, and develop questions in advance. In classes that require testing or a competency component (e.g., critical care classes, resuscitation classes, and skills-based teaching sessions), **Worksheets** can ensure readiness or provide a baseline for class awareness and mastery.
- If the material is complex, a **Worksheet** or handout can provide a framework for taking class notes and for studying later. If class material is difficult to understand, organizing it into a **Worksheet** may enable students to grasp it more easily.

All Things Being Equal

General Description   This strategy helps students learn to set priorities and to recognize signs and symptoms that may require more immediate attention. Students are given three or four different sets of signs and symptoms, lab data, or other client information. They're asked to rank the data according to level of acuity or priority and are given no additional information.

Frequently students want to know more details about the client or the circumstances of the case. This is where **All Things Being Equal** comes in. In this strategy, you tell the students that you've given them the most important data and ask them to base their decisions on that alone.

This strategy is a great help in developing test questions and enhancing critical thinking skills. Nursing students and nurses who take objective examinations often lament the need to rank four right answers to the same question. All are correct, but the test taker must identify the action of highest priority or the problem that needs the most urgent attention. **All Things Being Equal** develops the ability to make decisions based on limited amounts of information.

Preparation and Equipment   You can prepare this strategy easily while preparing a lecture or practicing your delivery. The exercises may be shown on an overhead or PowerPoint slide, as a handout, or on a blackboard.

Example of the Strategy at Work   I use **All Things Being Equal** to help students differentiate severe or life-threatening conditions from less urgent ones. During a lecture on pediatric respiration, the students needed to compare vital signs with norms, distinguish benign symptoms from more ominous ones, and interpret normal and abnormal lab data (Box 3–2). This strategy provided a framework in which they could practice their skills.

Because classes can bombard them with so much material, students may find it difficult to sift through and discern the signs and symptoms that take highest priority. Years of experience have taught practicing nurses the importance of keeping an airway patent, attending to physiological and safety needs, and managing pain. In contrast, novices find it difficult to sort data into levels of severity because they lack a clinical foundation for knowledge development. This strategy provides the perspective necessary for an informed nursing decision.

Ideas for Use

- Use **All Things Being Equal** to reinforce lab data. One difficult area for nursing students is the extent to which a lab result can deviate from the norm before it indicates a problem. For example, a practicing nurse knows the significance of a serum potassium level of 2.0 mEq/L, but a novice may not.
- You can base test questions on some of the exercises. Write a scenario for the test question and ask, "Which symptom concerns the nurse the most?" or "Which symptom indicates a need for immediate attention?"

Box 3–2.
Set Priorities for These Clients

(A) An infant with a respiratory rate of 18/min
(B) A school-age child with an expiratory wheeze
(C) A child with chronic allergies and an O_2 saturation of 90%

(A) An infant with a bobbing head
(B) An infant with peripheral cyanosis
(C) An adolescent with a barrel chest

(A) A child with bronchitis and coarse breath sounds
(B) An infant with slow seesaw respirations
(C) A child with asthma who has an intermittent cough

- Encourage students to quiz each other using **All Things Being Equal.** Making up these exercises is an excellent way for students to prepare for an examination.
- This strategy can be used to rank the priorities for several clients or to rank conflicting priorities in a single client. You can also ask questions about potential nursing interventions. This allows students to link assessments with interventions and provides a valuable skill often tested on NCLEX®.
- **All Things Being Equal** reinforces the need to set priorities and answer questions with only the information at hand. The student is forced to focus on limited but adequate amounts of data.

When You Think of This, Think of That

General Description   This strategy is a matching exercise used to reinforce classroom material. The information is set up in two columns, and students are asked to match items. It's important to have several correct matches; that way the students have to think rather than simply eliminate choices. Some items will have only one match, but others will have several. Box 3–3 shows an example: the only match for rheumatic heart disease is the sequela of an untreated streptococcal infection.

Preparation and Equipment   You'll need to set up your two-column list and decide the best way to present it. It can be made into a handout, put on an overhead or PowerPoint slide, or written on the blackboard. You can also use it as a format for **Quickie Quizzes** or **Quizzes that Count.**

Example of the Strategy at Work   In a pediatric respiration class I used a PowerPoint slide that the students could enlarge and use as a study aid. In class we discussed all the diagnoses in the right column and several items in the left column (see Box 3–3). We covered important concepts by focusing on the differences between gradual- and sudden-onset conditions. The strategy reinforced the importance of knowing the differences, and the students were able to practice the concepts in a matching exercise.

Ideas for Use

- Use **When You Think of This** for any subject matter in which students are asked to memorize or learn complex symptomatology or pathophysiology.
- This strategy can be adapted for **Quickie Quizzes** and **Quizzes that Count.**
- You can use the strategy in a game format: keep score, promote healthy competition, and give out prizes.

Box 3–3.
More Than One Answer Works

No intubation or throat examination	Epiglottis
"Barky" cough	Respiratory syncytial virus
Coughing, wheezing	Asthma
Pulling at ears	Bronchitis
High fever, drooling	Otitis media
Lots of nasal mucus	Tonsillitis
Sequelae—lack of strep medication	Acute nasal pharyngitis
Coarse breath sounds	Acute spasmodic laryngitis
Life-threatening situation	Acute laryngotracheal bronchitis
Medical and surgical management	Rheumatic heart disease
Bathroom shower	
Sudden onset	
Gradual onset	

- Encourage students to silently review lists used in **When You Think of This.** Then you can solicit answers. This tactic actively involves the students rather than letting them wait passively for answers without doing any work.

Current Events

General Description   In this strategy, current world events provide a springboard for class discussion or reinforce important concepts. Using a **Current Event** from the newspaper or television news can inspire up-to-date application of nursing knowledge. Students who are deeply embedded in schoolwork, or nurses who juggle several priorities, may be insulated from the goings-on of the world. However, nursing is a profession with a strong social conscience. This strategy introduces current affairs to the classroom and highlights the extent to which nursing can influence world situations.

Preparation and Equipment   Staying informed about current events is the only preparation needed for this strategy. Depending on the class objectives, **Current Events** may present themselves as major topics for discussion. Other news events may need to be researched by you or the students.

Example of the Strategy at Work   The following case summarizes a widely publicized event in which a family relinquished care of their disabled son. They pleaded stress and lack of respite resources. I used this case to discuss the stress of chronic illness on the family and their need for support to alleviate the constant demands of their son's condition.

A Current Case

A Family in Crisis

12/26: A mother allegedly drops off her disabled son, S., at a hospital, with a note stating that the parents could no longer care for him. S., who has cerebral palsy, is admitted to the hospital.

12/27: The parents surrender to police and are charged with child abandonment and conspiracy. These are misdemeanor charges.

12/28: The parents are released on condition that they have no contact with S.

12/29: Offers are made to watch S. The state would like to return him to his parents.

1/1: The father is given leave from work.

All current events should be presented as they were reported in the news, without editorial comment. If news is local, "insider" information should not be included. On the other hand, any news printed in a paper or aired on television is considered public record and appropriate for classroom discussion.

I've also used **Current Events** to update pharmacological information and present medical advances. Often the lay literature portrays a medical advance as a "breakthrough" and claims that it "abolishes" a condition. If in fact the story is based on a single research study or discovery, spirited classroom discussion may ensue. Such examples reinforce the need for a sound knowledge base before changes can be made in practice. What a great opportunity to teach this important principle of evidence-based practice.

Ideas for Use

- Students can be asked to provide the current event as part of a **Quick Write, E-mail Exercise,** or **Admit Ticket.**
- Most students remember the use of **Current Events** and will transfer their importance to higher education and the working world.

- Local health-related events also may be important to the class. Agency newsletters, community papers, or other resources may be used to access information.
- Students can use newspaper-related search engines (e.g., Lexus-Nexus) to conduct **Current Event** searches of subscribed works.

Bring In the Reinforcements and In-class Applications

General Description   This strategy requires a pause in your teaching so you can reinforce or apply concepts while they're being discussed. It's easy to gloss over material quickly without making sure the students understand it. **Bring In the Reinforcements** lets you use short class exercises to *reinforce* class material in a few moments. **In-class Applications** allows students to *apply* information quickly after hearing it. Both strategies increase the likelihood of learning and retention.

Preparation and Equipment   Develop the exercises after preparing your class material. These exercises should be short and to the point so the students can get immediate feedback about how well they've understood the concepts.

Example of the Strategy at Work   One way to **Bring In the Reinforcements** in class is to define terms and then ask students to identify examples. I use this tactic when discussing types of change: planned, developmental, covert, and so on. Then I show a slide listing selected examples of change (Boxes 3–4, 3–5). Students identify the types of change each example signifies, immediately reinforcing what they've just learned. The concept that more than one type of change may be applicable to life events is difficult and better explained with a concrete example.

An example of **Bring In the Reinforcements** comes from a continuing education program on assertiveness. Students were given a conflict common in their personal unit or job situation. They were asked to construct various responses: assertive, passive, aggressive, and passive-aggressive. Much as in **Invented Dialogues,** students not only practiced their constructed responses, but also compared the outcomes of each one in the given situation.

An example of **In-class Applications** is the use of mini-cases to apply

Box 3–4.
Types of Change

- Planned
- Unplanned
- Covert
- Overt
- Developmental
- More than one type

Box 3–5.
Types of Change

- A girl reaching puberty
- A teaching session on self-injection
- A toddler sustaining life-threatening burns by spilling scalding water
- A person gaining 50 lb
- Cancer growing in a 72-year-old woman's bones
- An 85-year-old having a cerebrovascular accident
- A nursing plan to help a client stop smoking
- A teaching session for new parents on baby care

concepts learned in class to "real-life" situations. One class focused on health and different individuals' reactions to illness. We discussed emotional dimensions, locus of control, external factors, and motivation. A brief case study revealed the stark differences between two clients' reactions to a heart attack. These cases illustrate the differences in clients' responses much better than a simple description would.

Applying Health Concepts

Jerry's Case
Jerry suffered a heart attack. On his physician's advice, he started exercising, changed his diet, entered stress management classes, and returned to work. He has a positive outlook and considers himself "well."

Joe's Case
After his heart attack, Joe also changed his diet and started exercising. However, he hasn't been able to quit smoking, although he wants to and has been vehemently advised to do so. Joe is often despondent and fears having another heart attack. He has not returned to work and describes himself as "ill."

Discussion Points

- Emotional dimensions
- Locus of control
- External factors
- Motivation
- Nursing interventions

Another way to use **In-class Applications** is to develop a short illustrative scenario and ask students to identify different features. I have used this method in teaching leadership styles. We discuss laissez-faire, autocratic, charismatic, and democratic styles. Then I lay the groundwork for the exercise.

Leadership Styles

You've progressed in your career and have recently become nurse leader of a nurse-run community health center. You recently became aware of a problem with long waits in the clinic. Clients are complaining about waiting 1½ hours for routine care and are starting to skip appointments. Realizing that the situation undermines the care the clinic provides, you begin to explore solutions.

I then show slides illustrating different leadership styles and ask the students to identify them (see following). I also tell them that they'll be expected to demonstrate their knowledge in future examination questions.

Name that Leadership Style I

You call a meeting with your staff. You appeal to their emotional side, reading them letters clients have written about their clinic experiences. The letters describe endless waits and sick children who go unattended. You discuss the personal impact of these long waits and suggest several solutions.
   What style is this?

Name that Leadership Style II

You call a meeting with your staff. You tell them the long waits are unacceptable. The clinic is coming up for grant renewal, and client satisfaction is an important parameter. You tell the staff they'll need to work faster, more efficiently, and with decreasing resources. You add that if conditions don't improve, heads will roll.
   What style is this?

Name that Leadership Style III

You call a meeting with your staff. You delineate the problem with long waits and ask the staff to solve it. Withholding any suggestions, you let the staff decide the best way to proceed. You ask them to come up with strategies and report back at the next meeting.

What style is this?

Name that Leadership Style IV

You call a meeting with your staff. Using a flipchart, you summarize the factors contributing to the long waits. You separate the staff into groups to find solutions to the most significant factors. Working with you, the groups will reconvene to discuss which solutions should be tried first.

What style is this?

Ideas for Use

- **Bring In the Reinforcements** and **In-class Applications** are great ways to review material before an examination.
- These strategies make good transitions to a different topic.
- These short cases make students aware of the importance of the material and the potential examination information.
- Experienced nurses may respond well to this strategy as a way to open class and remind them of information they've learned but perhaps forgotten. By applying basic concepts through a rein-forcing strategy, you can ensure that everyone is "on the same page" and ready to learn more advanced material.

Speak UP

General Description   Some students think of questions but don't always feel comfortable interrupting a lecture or creative strategy. That's where **Speak UP** comes in handy. If you say these two words at transitional points in the class, you give your students license to ask their questions or request that you repeat something. Simply pause at selected moments and say, **"Speak UP—this is your opportu-nity to ask questions or comment."** Instructors should emphasize that

Speak UP represents the students' time for individualized learning and growth.

Preparation and Equipment   The only preparation for this strategy is to review your plan for the class and create opportunities for questions. You can announce the question and answer period informally or use slides with the words **Speak UP**.

Example of the Strategy at Work   This strategy works in any class setting but is especially valuable in large classes. Sometimes students ask questions unthinkingly while taking notes; other questions demonstrate a lack of preparation for class. Sometimes such low-level questions frustrate other class participants. On the other hand, each student deserves some clarification of class material. By channeling questions to **Speak UP** periods, you give your students time to reflect on other students' questions and make sure they want to ask their own.

Ideas for Use

- This is a good strategy to use in large classes or when students have many questions. It allows material to flow while respecting students' needs for clarification.
- Many instructors don't wait long enough for students to compose their thoughts and questions. It's important to wait for a response after we say **Speak UP.** You can easily feel pressured to continue class, not allowing students a real opportunity to offer comments, questions, or observations.
- Gauge your time according to the needs of the entire class. This strategy does require you to exert some control to keep a few students from dominating the **Speak UP** time. Students with extensive needs may be invited to visit during office hours or to make an appointment to see you.
- **Speak UP** is a great test review. This strategy gives students a voice in the review session by encouraging them to ask questions and delineate areas of confusion. Rather than reverting to another lecture or teacher-led discussion, the test review is focused on the students' issues. In fact, tests reviews should be based on student questions and needs.
- This strategy is a great way to end a multi-session continuing education session or to segue from one class to the next. By saying "**Speak UP**" at the beginning or end of a class, you'll give participants the opportunity to seek additional information without interrupting the flow of the class.
- Questions that are closely aligned with class objectives can become **Think-Pair-Share, Teaching Trios,** or **Group Thought** exercises.

Quotation Pauses

General Description   I use chapter epigraphs throughout this book to reinforce material and to capture attention. Quotations provoke thought in the classroom and throw in a little entertainment. In this strategy, the instructor pauses at appropriate times and provides a quotation to reinforce or apply classroom concepts.

Preparation and Equipment   Simply have quotations available when material comes up. As with the chapter epigraphs, **Quotation Pauses** are meant to generate a "pause for thought" and provide a transition to new material.

Example of the Strategy at Work   I use this quotation to begin an adolescent health class:

> "Our youth now love luxury. They have bad manners, contempt for authority; they show disrespect for their elders and love chatter in place of exercise; they no longer rise when elders enter the room; they contradict their parents; chatter before company; gobble up their food and tyrannize their teachers."
>
> —Socrates, 5th century BC

By making the point that the "next generation" never really changes, this quotation puts generational differences in perspective. It also provides some humor to begin the class.

Ideas for Use

- Quotations can be found anywhere—newspapers, television, anthologies, calendars, inspirational posters, e-mail messages, colleagues, or daily life.
- Be attuned to quotations in your personal reading that could reinforce material or "grab" an audience.

Group Thought

General Description   Group work, or **Group Thought,** is a common strategy used in classrooms, large and small, to encourage interactive learning and active thinking. With **Group Thought,** groups of various sizes are directed to certain tasks. Each group may have the same task, or each may be given a different component of the assignment to report back to the larger class. By and large, students in academic classes look down on group activities as a distraction from testable material. In nonacademic settings, where participants are more receptive to passive learning, **Group Thought** may be considered frivolous and "not on task." Here are some hints to help you make **Group Thought** effective, objective driven, and productive.

Assigning Groups

For classroom activities, assigning groups is usually preferable to letting students pick their own.

- In large classes, group selection could take all day.
- Given the choice, friends tend to group together, which may not prove productive.
- Students who have a good grasp of the material tend to gravitate to others who also understand it. The converse is true: students who don't comprehend material choose to work with others who don't understand it.

Grouping Ideas

- Use the traditional "counting off" method: "One, two, three, four; one, two, three, four," and so on.
- Pass out fake money—distribute ones, fives, tens, twenties, and fifties. Ask the students with each denomination to find each other and form a group.
- Use colored pencils, birthday months, color of shirts, randomly picked numbers, or any other differentiating method.
- Use different types of candy to set up groups, with each class member trying to find a partner or group with the similar candy.
- Once groups are established, use them for one exercise or keep them together for future group work.

Preparation and Equipment   Prepare the exercise in advance. Ensure that it reinforces class content and meets your objectives. You may want to have supplies on hand to assist with group selection or prizes to hand out as rewards for participation in the exercise.

Example of the Strategy at Work   The most common **Group Thought** exercise is the case scenario with questions. All the groups are given the same questions and different cases. Students answer the questions in relation to the individual cases and then report back to the class.

I've used this type of exercise to reinforce legal and ethical principles in the classroom. Using an ethical decision-making model from their text, the groups of students review a case and answer these questions:

1. How would you respond?
2. What are the actual and potential legal issues?
3. What are the actual and potential impacts on ethical principles?

4. How do your values influence this scenario?
5. What could or should a nurse do, considering this information?

Here are some case studies I have used. Additional studies can be found online at http://davisplus.fadavis.com/herrman.

Case 1

A 50-year-old woman is admitted for uterine bleeding and pain. In the assessment, you discover that her husband died 1 week ago and that she is emotionally distraught. She meets with a surgeon who recommends a hysterectomy. The surgeon reviews the informed consent form rapidly and appears hurried. The client is distracted and inattentive, signing the consent form when urged to by the surgeon. You have watched the client–surgeon interaction, and the surgeon asks you to witness the consent.

Case 2

A client was admitted with lumbar disk herniation and placed in pelvic traction by a new graduate nurse. Although she had not performed the procedure before, she thought she could do it and did not check the hospital procedure manual. After 3 hours in traction, the client requested pain medication and removal of the traction.

The client noted that the IM injection did not hurt at all. He realized he had lost feeling in his buttocks and legs and became very agitated. He told the new nurse, who realized she had contributed to the problem. She was afraid to document the treatments and the new developments. She called the physician, who stated that disk herniation is frequently accompanied by these symptoms. The nurse was relieved and did not document the event. The client remained upset and refused traction. His numbness continued after hospitalization.

Case 3

At 7:30 a.m. a 60-year-old female postoperative client complains of pain. She states that she has not received pain medication since last night before bed. She wants to start her day with some pain medication on board. She appears alert and demonstrates signs and behaviors consistent with acute pain. When you review the medical review, you note that the narcotic pain medication was signed out at 8 p.m., 12 midnight, and 4 a.m. The client is due for medication at 8 a.m.

You wonder why the client does not remember the medication. When you look at her chart, you see no mention of medications or pain assessments. The night nurse did not mention administering pain medication, was sleepy in morning report, and expressed that she was anxious to go home.

Case 4

You are caring for a pediatric client receiving chemotherapy for leukemia. The chemotherapy is administered every 4 hr at 8 p.m. and 12 midnight on your evening shift. At 8 p.m. you are very busy with a heavy client assignment, many medications, and lots of treatments. You get your tasks done and feel accomplished in your abilities. At midnight, when you prepare the second dose of chemotherapy, you discover that you made a calculation error and gave double the dose at the 8 p.m. administration.

Case 5

A 75-year-old man is dying of lung cancer and is in extreme pain. You are a hospice nurse, visiting the client in his home. He lives alone and is grieving the loss of his wife 1 year ago. He expresses hopelessness and helplessness to you. He is in despair about his continued anguish and lack of relief. He asks you to leave him enough narcotic pain medication to allow him to self-administer a lethal dose. He is alert and has contemplated his choices. He is not asking you to administer the medication, just to provide enough so he can leave this world.

Students are asked to review these cases and answer the questions in a group. I keep the groups to three or four people to ensure that everyone participates. Because our classes are large, we frequently have more than one group per topic.

I ask each group to report to the class. Other groups add additional findings to the discussion. All the case studies can be found in the students' workbooks and may be used in a test. I instruct the students to review all the case studies and listen attentively in class in preparation for the examination.

Here's a **Group Thought** I've used with senior nursing students and practicing nurses. It involves delegation and how to decide patient assignments. These are difficult concepts to teach.

Management of Client Care: Case Study

The charge nurse is establishing the patient assignments for the shift. Here are the details of the clients and staff:

- Number of clients: 30
- Number of Registered Nurses: 4 plus the Charge Nurse
- Number of Unlicensed Assistive Personnel: 3

Here is the assignment for each Registered Nurse:

RN 1: 8 clients (all require routine care; 1 routine discharge)
RN 2: 6 clients (2 receiving blood; 1 new admission)
RN 3: 6 clients (1 complex discharge; 2 beginning chemotherapy)
RN 4: 8 clients (2 routine discharges; 1 recent postoperative client)
Charge Nurse: 2 clients (1 has a tracheostomy and is on a ventilator;
    1 needs routine care).

You are assigning the unlicensed assistive personnel (UAP) to assist in managing the unit. Here are the details for the care of the clients. Score them using the National Council of State Boards of Nursing Decision-making Grid, an assignment sheet from a local clinical agency, or one made up to reflect the data in the exercise.

Client 1: This client is being cared for by the charge nurse. He has been on a ventilator for 1 year secondary to cerebral anoxia following a cerebrovascular accident. The client needs lots of suctioning. He receives percutaneous endoscopic gastrostomy tube feedings and needs total care. The UAP is a senior nursing student who has cared for complex conditions but is not as familiar with ventilators. The charge nurse has 6 years' experience on the unit and is well versed in client care and delegation. The charge nurse has had the client the last two nights. The client's status is stable. He is incontinent and has a Glasgow Coma Scale score of 5. The UAP is asked to provide all a.m. care for the client.

Client 2: This client is under the care of RN 2. He has been newly admitted directly from the doctor's office. His diagnosis is COPD with acute exacerbation and mild respiratory distress. He is 89 years old and disoriented and has difficulty in swallowing. He needs assistance with activities of daily living and ambulation; he can wash and feed himself. The UAP has been on the unit for 3 years and typically cares for clients with similar needs. The RN caring for the client has been pulled from the pediatric unit but is experienced in the care of clients with respiratory distress. The UAP is asked to provide all a.m. care for the client.

Client 3: This client is under the care of RN 3. She is postoperative, having had open-heart surgery. She was transferred yesterday from the cardiovascular intensive care unit after being treated for cardiogenic shock and ventricular dysrhythmias. She has a chest tube hooked to 20-cm wall suction through a Pleur-evac device. She is receiving 40 percent oxygen through a Venturi mask. She is at high risk for postoperative ventricular rhythm disturbances. The RN assigned to the client has had a telemetry course and has moderate experience with cardiac rhythms and postoperative cardiac care. The UAP has recently finished orientation and has not worked with the cardiovascular surgical population. The UAP is asked to provide all a.m. care for the client.

Students are divided into groups. They're given a copy of the National Council of State Boards of Nursing Decision-making Grid (available in many texts and at www.ncsbn.org). This assignment is an excellent one but does take 15 minutes to complete, potentially taking time from other activities.

Ideas for Use

- Stay in the classroom and roam among the groups. An instructor who leaves the room, checks voice mail, or does other work communicates to the class that the activity is not very entertaining or of much value for participants.
- When students move into groups, allow them to be comfortable. Let them sit on the floor, turn chairs, or leave the room if that's possible.
- Keep group activities short—5 to 7 minutes—and keep time carefully. Difficult or in-depth assignments may prove daunting, and the groups may spend more time complaining than working.

- Set clear time parameters for **Group Thought.** Use whistles or other attention-getting devices to call the class to order. You may want the students to stay in their positions or return to their more traditional seating patterns when the groups report or when class resumes.
- You may want to vary the size of the groups or their composition. This tactic is helpful if groups aren't staying on task or if one group appears to be struggling more than another.
- For academic classes, make sure that the students connect the group activity with class objectives and testable material.
- Listen to the volume of the group activities. Experience has taught me that the volume in the room goes up when the groups finish their task and revert to personal conversation. Give 1-minute warnings and roam around the room to ensure that groups stay on task.
- **Group Thought** is a great way to foster cooperative learning of complex material, such as setting priorities; interpreting lab, ECG, or arterial blood gas data; determining methods of conflict resolution; or focusing on important nursing interventions related to client needs, as in the perioperative period.
- **Group Thought** is an important strategy for building rapport among nurses who work together or spend time together between units. Case studies that reflect clinical skills and daily nursing practice are well received.

Using Mnemonics

General Description We use mnemonics throughout our lives to remember facts. They provide verbal cues to remembering complex or difficult information. This is an area in which students and instructors can share their "memory devices" with each other.

Preparation and Equipment The only preparation for this strategy is to remind yourself to **Use Mnemonics** when covering class content.

Example of the Strategy at Work Students have great ideas about mnemonics, and experience allows us all to accumulate them as we go along. Here are a few I enjoy:

In a class on neurological deterioration I explain decorticate and decerebrate posturing. I tell the class that in decorticate posturing the client brings the upper extremities "toward the core." The word "decerebrate" has more Es, indicating extension of the arms.

When we discuss the uses of different antigout medications, students learn about allopurinol and colchicine. Allopurinol is given for chronic gout and colchicine for acute gout, so I tell the students that the As and Cs don't match up.

In the class on diabetes, I tell students that hypoglycemia is the "wet one," marked by diaphoresis, and that hyperglycemia is the "dry one," with symptoms of dehydration.

The ABCs of the alphabet are used to reinforce Airway–Breathing–Circulation concepts in cardiopulmonary resuscitation. When memorizing the steps of the nursing process, students are taught to think of "A Delicious Apple PIE" to remember Assessment, Diagnosis–Analysis, Planning, Implementation, and Evaluation. The potential list is endless. The importance of this strategy is the ability of students to make their own connections and to understand and **Use Mnemonics** consistently.

Ideas for Use

- Try to **Use Mnemonics** any time a complex process requires some level of memorization.
- Several published memorization resources can provide additional ideas. Go to www.medicalmnemonics.com to access additional mnemonics for nursing education.
- Have students post their "memory tools" on the class Web site or in **Online Discussions.**
- Make sure students understand that mnemonics are memory devices and that they'll eventually need to step beyond retention to critical thinking. Memorization allows students to move on and think more analytically and critically about memorized material.
- Use the strategy of metaphor much as you would use mnemonics. One instructor based the entire class on a "recipe for success" and referred frequently to cooking, ingredients, time, and the product to build a story for the class participants.

Keep 'em Awake Quizzes, Quickie Quizzes, Quizzes that Count

General Description   Just the mention of the word "quiz" makes students sit up straighter, complain, and panic. From the perspective of the instructor, quizzes provide a valuable way to assess understanding, document class attendance, and get a continuous measure of preparation and knowledge acquisition. Not all quizzes have to count, but quizzes interspersed with classroom presentations may provide a useful way to assess learning.

Keep 'em Awake Quizzes are simply two or three questions asked in the middle of class. They let you assess understanding and get a "read" on the class. **Quickie Quizzes** can be used as an opener to refresh previously learned material or reinforce preparation for that day's class. These two types of quiz don't count toward the course grade but can be effectively used in continuing education and staff development. **Quizzes that Count** can assess class knowledge, encourage participation and preparation, and offer another chance to students whose test grades are low because of anxiety or poor performance. For our purposes, quizzes consist of three to eight questions and take up less than 10 minutes of class time.

Preparation and Equipment   Write the quiz and the answer key before class. Set aside class time for the quiz—you may provide the answers right after the quiz or later. For **Quizzes that Count,** make sure the quiz policy is clear in the class syllabus and that there are guidelines for quiz make-ups and grading. You can hand out quizzes or put them on regular or PowerPoint slides. For quiz handouts, use colored paper to make sure students hand them in, or half sheets to conserve paper.

Example of the Strategy at Work

Quickie Quiz

For a class opener, I've asked students complete the following quiz. Our curriculum teaches pathophysiology separately from nursing interventions. As a way to remind students about what they've already learned, I start the class with this quiz. The students are always told, "It doesn't count!"

Quickie Quiz

Cystic Fibrosis Quiz—It Doesn't Count!

1. CF is marked by _____ gland dysfunction.

2. CF is inherited as a _____ trait.

3. The mucus produced in CF can be described as _____ and _____.

4. Stagnant respiratory mucus leads to _____, _____, and _____.

5. Fibrotic changes in the pancreas prevent the release of _____ into the _____.

6. Stools containing fat (_____) and protein (_____) are found in clients with CF.

7. Respiratory assessment of a client with CF and significant pulmonary involvement would show _____.

8. Respiratory care includes _____.

Keep 'em Awake Quizzes

In the middle of class I show a few questions on slides to determine how well the students comprehend the material (see following).

Keep 'em Awake Quiz

The nurse is caring for a client with a laryngectomy for whom all of the following actions are necessary. Which action should take priority?
  A. Bathing and hygiene
  B. Assisting with breakfast
  C. Suctioning the airway
  D. Ambulating to the bathroom

Which of the following is an intervention to prevent the most common complication of a splenectomy?
  A. Ambulation
  B. Coughing and deep breathing
  C. Maintaining IV fluids
  D. Isolation precautions

Asking these questions allows students to apply material immediately and show whether or not they understand it.

Quizzes that Count

This strategy was shared with me by a colleague who attended a conference on student evaluation. Participants had complained about poor class attendance, lack of preparation, and lack of attentiveness. **Quizzes that Count** were developed as a result of these frustrations. They consist of three questions: the student's name (as a way to take attendance), one about the class readings, and one about the class discussion.

Following is the quiz I give in the middle of the class on cleft lip and palate. At the time I've discussed cleft lip but not cleft palate, so the second question assesses attentiveness and the third question the level of class preparation.

A Quiz That Counts

1. Name: _____
2. Name one nursing intervention to protect the incision after a cleft lip repair.
3. Name one nursing intervention to protect the incision after a cleft palate repair.

We allot points in each student's grade for these quizzes. They're given randomly throughout the semester and are unannounced. It's best to vary the time to ensure that the class attends the entire session.

Our faculty has embraced these quizzes with some controversy. Many believe that class attendance and preparation are a personal choice and a component of adult learning. For more junior students, however, quizzes provide structure and incentive to attend and illustrate the importance of class readiness. We drop one quiz per semester from the grade to allow for unexcused absences. Our policy is conservative in what we consider an excused absence.

Ideas for Use

- Develop a **Keep 'em Awake Quiz** in a class with complex material before moving on to the next topic. Students may not admit they don't know something—or haven't even thought about it yet. A small quiz will highlight the material and allow students to figure out whether they "get it" or have any questions.
- These **Quizzes** may be used for extra credit when student interest is waning, as before breaks or at the end of the semester.
- **Quizzes** may be used in continuing education programs, such as critical care or other classes in which students are expected to review before attending.
- Use **Quizzes** to focus studying for examinations, or give them before class to ensure that students are prepared. You'll reward their preparation by just going over the answers in class or in a review session.
- **Quizzes** are a great way to keep attention in a continuing education or staff development class. Prizes or other incentives can make them even more interesting.
- Use old examination questions for **Quizzes** to get students comfortable with the level of difficulty and the test question format. You can "recycle" old quiz questions for subsequent examinations. Doing this reinforces the importance of class attendance.
- Using **Quickie Quizzes** at the beginning of class encourages students to be on time and settle in quickly.

Feedback Lecture

General Description   The **Feedback Lecture** is a well-documented strategy used to complement traditional lectures. Osterman[11] developed this method as a means of combining lecture with performance-based instruction. In this way, feedback becomes reciprocal, with both students and teachers learning throughout the process.

As originally designed, the **Feedback Lecture** includes procedures, an introduction, objectives, a pretest, an outline, discussion questions, feedback on discussion questions, warm-up activities, and a post-test. Because I've adapted this method to allow for quick feedback, my method includes a pretest, the standard test outline, and a post-test. I encourage you to research the **Feedback Lecture** and use it in any form useful to your own teaching needs.

Preparation and Equipment   As originally designed, this method does take a fair amount of preparation. Even for the abridged version you need to develop the pretest, outline the lecture (usually done anyway), write the lecture (necessary), and develop the post-test. Once the work is done, however, the **Feedback Lecture** can be used repeatedly in classes.

Example of the Strategy at Work

Pretest

1. Name three components of the preoperative check that the nurse is responsible for completing before sending a client into surgery.
2. Name three components of preoperative teaching and three common postoperative complications that can be prevented through preoperative teaching.
3. Name one way to confirm a client's identity before a surgical procedure.
4. Discuss three differences between the scrub nurse and the circulating nurse.

Discussion Questions

1. How do you respond when you believe a client does not comprehend his or her preoperative teaching?
2. How would you react in the operating room if you were in a situation where a client's condition deteriorated?
3. What safety factors are in place to ensure that the correct surgery is done on a client?
4. How would you react to an immediately postoperative client who refuses pain medication?

Class Outline

I. The role of the nurse in the care of the preoperative client

    A. Preoperative assessments
    B. Preoperative teaching
    C. Safety and risk management

II. The role of the nurse in the care of the intraoperative client

    A. The circulating nurse and the scrub nurse
    B. Anesthesia agents, stages, and client responses
    C. Estimated blood loss; estimated blood replaced

III. The role of the nurse in caring for the postoperative client

    A. Assessments and monitoring
    B. Postanesthesia care unit parameters
    C. Postoperative complications and prevention
    D. Pain and pain management
    E. Diet and activity progression
    F. Dressings and drains
    G. IV therapy
    H. Transfer to the unit or discharge
    I. Discharge teaching

I have used this method to teach difficult topics with many different facets, such as perioperative nursing. I provide the pretest, give the short lecture, allow group discussion on several questions, and then give the post-test. I use the same pre- and post-test for this exercise, but you can make up different ones. We allot significant time to the lecture and discussion portions, encouraging the students to do the pretest before class and the post-test as an **E-mail Exercise.**

Ideas for Use

- Intersperse **Group Thought** with the **Feedback Lecture** to combine lecture content with interactive learning.
- Use the **Feedback Lecture** with **Admit Ticket** and allow the pretest to be the student's "entrance fee" into class.
- Develop the **Feedback Lecture** format for each class so students get into the habit of being prepared and completing the pretest before class. Build on the pretest questions to construct examination questions.
- For small classes, have individuals or groups develop classes, class outlines, and pre- and post-tests. They can present class content to each other while you reinforce or clarify information.
- Use textbook resources to develop pre- and post-test questions and class outlines.
- Refer to the resources in the Annotated Bibliography for more details about using the **Feedback Lecture** in your classroom.

References

1. Herrman, J: Using film clips to enhance nursing education. Nurse Educator 31(6):264–269, 2006.
2. Weeks, CS: Text-Book for Nursing. Appleton & Co, New York, 1885.
3. Chenovert, M: What Do Nurses Do? Pro-Nurse, Gaithersburg, MD, 2000.
4. Buscaglia, L: The Fall of Freddy the Leaf. Holt Rinehart & Winston, 1983.
5. Moss, J: Bob and Jack A Boy and his Yak. Bantam, New York, 1992.
6. Scieszka, J: The True Story of the Three Little Pigs. Scholastic, New York, 1989.
7. Jackson, K: Nurse Nancy. Golden Books, New York, 1952.
8. Gaspard, H: Doctor Dan the Bandage Man. Golden Books, New York 1950.
9. Bond, E: Remembering Nancy Nurse. A nurse educator reflects upon a powerful childhood role model. Reflections on Nursing Leadership 28(4):8–9, 2002.
10. Glendon, KJ, and Ulrich, DL: Unfolding Case Studies: Experiencing the Realities of Clinical Nursing Practice. Prentice-Hall, Upper Saddle River, NJ, 2001.
11. Osterman, D: Feedback Lecture Idea Paper #13. Kansas State University, Manhattan, KS, 1985.

Chapter 4

Strategies for Small Classes

"Implementing creative teaching strategies that will change a classroom from a four-walled room with educational hopes into an environment that is infused with excitement, curiosity, and genuine student learning." —Joseph S.C. Simplicio

Challenges

- Small classes are usually the most enjoyable to teach. Many instructors feel at their most effective when working with a group of this size. Still, small classes present challenges in reaching all the students. Their size varies. In some situations a class of 10 is considered small; in others, a small class can comprise as many as 50 students. Generally the strategies in this chapter are useful for groups of 20 to 30, although subtle changes can adapt them to bigger or smaller classes.

- Some students are reluctant to participate and may feel conspicuous in the smaller classroom because it lacks the anonymity of larger classes.

- Smaller classes may be graded for participation. Some contributions are more valuable than others and some students do not actively participate in class. Therefore, assessing a student's participation creates special challenges for the instructor.

- Small classrooms are especially vulnerable to group dynamics. The personality of the class may encourage a spirit of inquiry or its negative counterpart, a spirit of disdain. Group cohesiveness, or its lack, may challenge instructors who wish to engage students in active strategies.

- Smaller classes may need considerable teaching energy to maintain a high pace of learning and zest for more information.

Small classes offer a great environment for cooperative learning, problem-based formats, and group learning strategies. Creative teaching strategies can enhance an already fertile ground for learning. Innovative teaching gives the instructor a chance to assess group attitudes and needs and improve group functioning. If you're teaching a small class, you can use creative strategies to provide one of the most pleasurable learning experiences for yourself and your students.

IDEAS

Six Hats Exercise

General Description   The Six Thinking Hats activity was originally developed by deBono[1] as a way to encourage team building and conflict resolution. Gross[2] has used this tool with nurses and health-care workers to cultivate decision-making, teamwork, and empathy.

In this exercise, hats of different colors represent different ways of looking at an issue. Participants are given hats, each representing a different perspective on an issue. Each student is asked to view a situation through the assigned color. Gross[2] uses the colored hats to represent different perspectives including red (emotional), green (creative), black (pessimistic), white (logical), yellow (optimistic), and blue (overarching values). Figure 4–1 shows possible interpretations of the six hats and the perspective each represents.

Preparation and Equipment   If you wish to use this technique, you'll need a situation that lends itself to debate and different perspectives. Look for color-appropriate party hats or other toy hats to pass out to each member of the team. If class size permits, each group should have six members.

Example of the Strategy at Work   I've used this strategy to work on problem-solving skills in two different situations. In the first, a nursing clinical group had just met each other several days before. They encountered a client in circumstances similar to those described in Box 4–1. The students, seeing an ethical issue firsthand, were having a difficult time resolving it both within and among themselves. I used the **Six Hats Exercise** to get them thinking about their own personal views, the perspectives of others, and how to use problem-solving skills in a true dilemma.

In post-conference I passed out six sheets of colored paper, corresponding to the colors of the hats. My group had seven people, so I gave two people a blue sheet. One person acted as recorder and another as moderator. I set the ground rules for the discussion and the exercise began.

The "blue hat" started the conversation and asked each "hat" to address the situation from its perspective. After each member contributed to the

THE SIX HATS

Emotional	Overarching Values	Logical
Creative	Optimistic	Pessimistic

Fig. 4–1.   Different perspectives provide a forum for discussion.

conversation, the entire group discussed the ethical problem. The students analyzed the issue using their new understanding and perspectives.

During an in-service training for faculty members, I used the exercise shown in Box 4–2. In this setting, the point of the exercise was to demonstrate its versatility and its possible use in many conflict situations. It's a great decision-making guide and an effective icebreaker. You can use it in

---

Box 4–1.
Six Hats for Clinical Nursing Students

Your group has been caring for a client with a ventilator for 1 month. Each member of your group has cared for the client at least once. The client is unresponsive except to painful stimuli and is displaying decerebrate posturing. Sustenance is maintained by the ventilator, hydration, and nasogastric tube feedings.

The students are feeling conflicted, especially because the family keeps asking when the client will be better and able to go home. The medical ethics committee has recommended discontinuing the ventilator. Use the six hats to address this issue.

Box 4–2.
Six Hats for Faculty Members

You have a clinical group with eight juniors. Three have worked as hospital aides and two are second-career adult learners. The group has a considerable amount of discord, poor teamwork skills, and a low level of motivation. They bicker and compete with each other. As the instructor, you realize something has to be done. As a group of faculty, use the six hats to come up with potential solutions to resolve the group dysfunction.

leadership training as a strategy for dealing with difficult situations and understanding other perspectives.

Ideas for Use

- Faculty may find **Six Hats** a great strategy to use in legal and ethical discussions, with clinical groups, or any time a sensitive issue needs to be addressed.
- Instead of hats, you can give students color-coded name tags.
- Use the **Six Hats Exercise** when conflicts exist or when team work is otherwise a challenge. This exercise builds rapport and collegiality. It also develops empathy skills by challenging participants to understand points of view different from their own.
- If time permits, have participants wear more than one hat so they can view a situation from multiple perspectives.
- If you know the group well, assign colors that don't fit the participants' characteristic personalities. For example, give the eternal pessimist a yellow hat and the unemotional person a red one. Arguing from an unaccustomed position fosters critical thinking skills.
- After all the participants have expressed their views, use the discussion time for debriefing. Analyze not only the situation, but also the group process. Talk about the emotions and the knowledge participants glean from "walking in each others' moccasins."
- Combine **In-Class Debate** with **Six Hats.** Your students will combine research with the perspectives of others to address common issues and arrive at workable conclusions.

In-basket Exercise

General Description   The **In-basket Exercise,** first described by Sweeney and Moeller,[3] gives students a task, a time frame, and a limited amount of information. This strategy is a lot like getting an assignment in your in-basket. Decisions need to be made based on this information as it comes to the in-basket, potentially without the opportunity to solicit additional information or view the situation from a variety of perspectives. These exercises are effective in developing group cohesiveness, as early group activities, and in helping students solve problems with incomplete information.

Preparation and Equipment   You need to develop case scenarios that relate to class objectives. The **In-basket Exercise** works on priority setting, group process, and conflict resolution.

The group solves a problem using only the data presented. Each group receives a case study that articulates the client's needs. The case study provides just enough information to ensure resolution, but not enough to allow for significant deliberation about the work. Case scenarios may be tailored to specific class content and class objectives.

Example of the Strategy at Work   Here is the exercise I give in class. The students need to base decisions on the information given to them—no extraneous information will be provided—so I issue the following warning:

> This exercise will assist you in analyzing group process. You will have 10 minutes to work in groups of six. All groups will work on the same issue, so it will be interesting to see how different groups think. We will reconvene for 5 minutes to discuss your results and rationales. I'll ask you then to consider the group process information we've have discussed in class. We'll assess how your group functioned, the patterns of decision-making, and the leadership styles.

The exercise follows:

Stuck

You work in a building with 10 floors. The six group members are on an elevator going up when the elevator stops. When you call for help, you find that all six passengers must be stuck on the elevator for 24 hours. There is no immediate threat to your safety, but you will not be able to get out.

The security manager will be able to send down one 20-in × 20-in × 20-in cardboard carton of supplies for your group to use in those 24 hours. This is all you are allowed. The elevator has ample room and there is enough oxygen for the duration. The security manager will contact you in 10 minutes to determine your requests. Please include a brief rationale for each supply item.

After the group work, it's beneficial to share findings within the class. Repeated use of this strategy teaches the common needs of existence (a great way to reinforce Maslow's Hierarchy of Needs[4]) but also highlights the individuality of human needs. Hygiene, water, food, and diversional activities are paramount. More technical needs—medication, blood glucose monitors, or sedation for people with claustrophobia—enlighten group members to the varied needs of others. This exercise also highlights the complexities of disaster and emergency management.

I used the strategy in a continuing education seminar as a light-hearted exercise for determining the contents of an emergency code bag. Participants in an advanced life support conference were given the following task. As you can imagine, a spirited discussion followed this assignment:

You are a transport person who is asked to stock a box with the supplies needed for emergency resuscitation and transport. Unfortunately you can only take enough supplies to fit a 10-in × 18-in × 24-in bag. Spend the next 10 minutes deciding the integral components for that emergency response bag.

Ideas for Use

- Subjects for **In-basket Exercises** may come from clinical situations, legal and ethical conflicts, priority setting, conflicts, and other nursing situations.

- For this strategy to succeed, the group must understand that no more information is available. Like our in-basket, these exercises provide only what's there without the luxury of other details.

- You can follow the **In-basket Exercise** with a class discussion or use a **Write to Learn** or **Quick Write** as an opportunity to comment. **Ah-hah Journals** may also be used to reflect on the exercise.

- **In-basket Exercises** can keep pace with the increasing knowledge base of a student or novice nurse. You can make the strategy more complex by including more detail about client conditions and clinical situations. This exercise is feasible at many levels of practice. You simply need to design it so students can answer the questions while continuing to feel challenged.

- Carefully constructed **In-basket Exercises** provide a great vehicle for any nursing lesson involving selected data, conflicting priorities, and the establishment of key concerns.

- Orientees may do an **In-basket Exercise** to learn to deal with nurse-physician conflicts, reacting in sensitive situations, delegating, and other simulated situations.

The Right Thing To Do

General Description   **The Right Thing To Do** is a particularly good way to introduce legal and ethical issues. This strategy helps to socialize beginning nurses and nursing students. Hypothetical cases, real issues, or potential dilemmas are presented in class. Students are then asked, "What is **The Right Thing To Do**?"

Preparation and Equipment   Anticipate when legal and ethical issues will come into the foreground of class discussion. Make notations in your lecture notes to set time aside for these issues.

Example of the Strategy at Work   In a discussion about the rights associated with participation in research, such as informed consent, justice, autonomy, and risks versus benefits, I presented several ethical questions to the students (see following). After reading each one I asked, "What is **The Right Thing To Do**?"

Asking individual students this question encourages the entire class to stay involved in the process. Applying the question in different circumstances will stimulate the development of both critical thinking and professional valuing. I presented the following situations:

- You discover that a colleague has been taking supplies from the unit closet and taking them home for personal use. What is **The Right Thing To Do?**
- A client is very worried that she will undergo the wrong surgical procedure. What is **The Right Thing To Do?**
- A colleague comes to work dressed unprofessionally. What is **The Right Thing To Do?**
- You are caring for a child in the hospital. Walking into the room, you find the child's mother hitting the child repeatedly. What is **The Right Thing To Do?**
- The wife of your client's roommate asks you about the health status of your client. What is **The Right Thing To Do?**

This strategy can promote discussion of some of the general knowledge aspects of nursing. Ask students to reflect on interventions from the commonsense viewpoint inherent in nursing care. Nursing instructors have been accused of stripping innate knowledge from people with common sense, then filling their brains with "nursing knowledge." At any level, this exercise helps instructors recapture the students' common sense and encourage the students to think before acting.

A good example happened with a student I taught early in my educational career. The student had four children; I had none and was fresh out of my graduate program. One evening in clinical the student rushed toward me in a panic. A child she was taking care of had a temperature of 39.5 degrees Celsius.

The student asked, "Judy, what do we do?" in a panicked voice. I replied, "What would you do if you were home and one of your children had that body temperature?" In essence I was asking her, "What is **The Right Thing To Do?**" She answered that she would force fluids, take off excess blankets, give an antipyretic, and call the doctor. I responded, "That's what we do here," indicating that we used the same measures in the clinical area to address a fever.

A component of nursing education is the license to use thinking skills and common sense in solving problems. **The Right Thing To Do** provides that opportunity.

Ideas for Use

- Use a legal and ethical decision-making framework to expand the strategy. In class you can share this strategy with the students. Then provide students with legal or ethical case studies such as those that follow and then simply ask, "What is **The Right Thing To Do?**

Case 1

A 20-year-old male client reveals during a database completion that he has been a prostitute for 4 years and has engaged in homosexual and heterosexual relationships. He is admitted with signs of respiratory and GI infections and is undergoing diagnostic procedures to pinpoint the origin of the infections. He asks you not to tell anyone and becomes angry and anxious over his divulging this information.

Case 2

An 18-year-old female client was given general anesthesia for the reduction and casting of fractures of her tibia and fibula. As she was waking up from anesthesia, the nurse explained her care following discharge while her friend went to get the car for the trip home. The nurse charted, "Client was instructed and discharged in a wheelchair with her friend." The client went home to bed, took her pain medication, and fell asleep. She awoke finding her foot swollen, cold, and bluish. She attributed these signs and her increasing pain to the fall that caused the fractures. Three days later, she was admitted to the hospital and required a below-the-knee amputation.

Case 3

A 76-year-old woman from a nursing home is admitted to an acute care facility in acute dehydration. The woman's usual mentation is disorganized but alert. The dehydration has caused her to be disoriented and combative. Restraints are applied to maintain her safety and prevent her from pulling out her intravenous lines. She is visited by her daughter, who is very upset about the restraints. The daughter contends that her mother's nursing home is a restraint-free environment and asks that the restraints be removed.

Case 4

You are an RN supervising nursing assistants. At the beginning of your shift, you discover that one of the clients has been experiencing dizziness and complaining of lightheadedness. When you delegate tasks to the nursing assistant, you instruct her to be cautious when helping the client to walk. You encourage her to seek out help if needed. At 10 p.m. the nursing assistant comes to tell you that she found the client on the bathroom floor. She states that she left the client at the sink to brush her teeth while she saw to another client's needs. The client is sitting on the bathroom floor holding her head when you arrive.

Case 5

A 45-year-old man is a client in your community clinic. He has a known history of drug abuse and has been treated recently for a fractured femur. He arrives at the clinic complaining of continued pain. The physician orders you to dispense a placebo medication, arguing that the client is addicted to the drugs and is not experiencing real pain.

Case 6

You work in a family planning clinic. You are completing the database for a 16-year-old girl who believes she is pregnant. You find that she has one 3-year-old child and has had two abortion procedures since the birth of that child. Her pregnancy test is negative, but you find that she has been forced to have sexual relations with her older brother's friends.

Ideas for Use

- Asking "What is **The Right Thing to Do?**" encourages students to use common sense and basic principles to reason through a situation.
- Bowles[5] proposed a game entitled "Find the Error." In this exercise, instructors provide statements with incorrect components. Students correct the statements using critical thinking skills. These statements are meant to challenge analytical skills rather than simple recall of facts.
- This strategy may be used to discuss any legal or ethical dilemma, including substance abuse, access to care, and much more.
- Discussing **The Right Thing To Do** is a great way to spark conversation in the clinical area. Frequently students feel pulled between the priorities of clinical work, the needs of the client, and whatever conflicts their classes have taught them to anticipate. The strategy challenges students to consider several perspectives and come to some conclusion about what is and isn't right.
- Clinical groups may discuss nursing practices different from the ones they've learned previously. This exercise helps them judge the merits and the rightness of unfamiliar practices.
- Students have trouble accepting the fact that different methods can produce the same result. They want to learn the one right method and are frustrated by multiple perspectives. **The Right Thing To Do** emphasizes that many things can be done in more than one way.
- The strategy reminds nurses of their responsibility for ensuring the basic principles of asepsis, safety, and client respect. Any alternative method must adhere to these principles. The old adage "There's more than one way to skin a cat" reinforces the reality of multiple approaches in many nursing processes. A discussion of basic principles can go a long way toward allaying fears and clarifying procedures, and may generate research questions about clinical practice.

Gaming

General Description   Any nursing class content can be put into game format. You can choose a marketed game, adapt a game show, or devise your own games at home.

Preparation and Equipment   When planning a game, keep in mind the class objectives, group size, and volume of content. Games can last 10 minutes or the entire class period. You can use them to test knowledge or provide an unusual out-of-class study. You may want to clarify the purpose of the game—teaching information, reinforcing content, assessing knowledge level, summarizing a class, or reviewing for an examination.

In smaller classes you can use board games to teach concepts. These games can be purchased or you can make your own. You can also adapt a game show to assist with course-specific content. Students enjoy the competition, creativity, and fun associated with gaming in the classroom, but the games do take a lot of preparation and time in the classroom.

One game show popular in the classroom is *Jeopardy*. You need to pick the topic for *Jeopardy*, finding five categories for answers. You compose five answers for each category in which questions are progressively more difficult as the money amount increases on the chart. Some instructors choose to develop a "daily double" to add an extra challenge.

Example of the Strategy at Work   Table 4–1 shows my game board for *Developmental Jeopardy*. I use this game to teach the developmental aspects of caring for a client with diabetes. PowerPoint lets me use animation in my game boards, and I can make answers emerge with a mouse click. The more real you can make the game, the better.

Developmental Jeopardy

In *Developmental Jeopardy* I use some of the following questions for the Cognitive Understanding category:

100 This developmental skill allows children to use literature, check doses, and use lists.

(What is reading?)

200 This developmental skill allows school-age children to categorize the symptoms of hyperglycemia and hypoglycemia.

(What is classification?)

Table 4–1. Developmental Jeopardy

Psychomotor Skills	Psychoemotional Characteristics	Cognitive Understanding	Teaching Strategies	Name that Stage
100	100	100	100	100
200	200	200	200	200
300	300	300	300	300
400	400	400	400	400
500	500	500	500	500

300 This developmental skill allows school-age children to know when to get injections, snacks, and meals.

(What is the concept of time?)

400 An adolescent girl needs to know that during her menses, insulin needs may_____.

(What is increase?)

500 This form of reasoning allows children to make the leap from signs and symptoms of hypoglycemia to action steps.

(What is inductive?)

Here's an example of the questions I use for the *Teaching Principles* category:

100 Doing an activity over and over adheres to this principle of teaching skills.

(What is repetition?)

200 Using a doll could assist in teaching these skills.

(What are insulin administration and blood glucose monitoring?)

300 These strategies may be effective in teaching diet planning to school-age children.

(What are meal planning and 24-hour diet recall?)

400 Including the family is an effective teaching strategy because diabetes is this kind of disease.

(What is a family disease?)

500 Role playing may be effective in addressing emotional issues because it does this.

(What is provides practice or develops empathy?)

In this class, *Jeopardy* is used to introduce the content. When you use a game to teach a topic for the first time, make sure the content is easily understood or that it synthesizes existing knowledge. You can also provide a **Worksheet** or handout for students who need more comprehensive and organized coverage of the topic.

My favorite use of *Jeopardy* is in test reviews. Students seem to especially enjoy *Pharmacology Jeopardy* as a way to prepare for the final examination. I bring bells for the students to ring when they have an answer and give prizes to everyone. I'm always surprised at the level of competition these games create, even though no real rewards or consequences are associated with them.

Gaming doesn't have to get this elaborate to be fun and thought-provoking. Puzzles and simple games make great brain teasers and icebreakers; on the first day of clinical rotation they help to allay fears and encourage teamwork. Here is one inspired by a common household magazine.

Rhyming Puzzlers

Think of a three-word common phrase to rhyme with the Puzzler.

Puzzler	**Answers**
1. Took, Sign, Blinker	Hook, Line, Sinker
2. Flop, Cook, Glisten	Stop, Look, Listen
3. Leg, Sorrow, Wheel	Beg, Borrow, Steal
4. Trap, Shackle, Top	Snap, Crackle, Pop
5. Mud, Fret, Cheers	Blood, Sweat, Tears
6. Sprawl, Tedium, Barge	Small, Medium, Large
7. Ball, Stark, Ransom	Tall, Dark, Handsome
8. Versed, Beckoned, Heard	First, Second, Third
9. Wife, Pork, Croon	Knife, Fork, Spoon
10. Head, Fright, Crew	Red, White, Blue

Match Game

Another game I used is much simpler and makes a good icebreaker. I gave each student an index card. Half the cards listed the major signs and symptoms of a disease or condition; the other half had the names of those diseases or conditions. Students had to travel around the room to find the card that matched theirs. The game took only 5 minutes, yet provided a rapid review of class content. Box 4–3 shows some of the Match Game cards I used when teaching newborn assessment.

Ideas for Use

- **Gaming** is a great way for both you and your students to assess knowledge before class discussion or in preparation for an examination.

- Use **Gaming** at the end of the semester, or the end of the course, as an examination review or to encourage cumulative learning.

- There are several marketed games developed by entrepreneurial nurses to foster learning. One such individual is Kathleen Walsh Free, who developed a game called *"What if? What else? What then?"*[6] Free has developed more than eight games to reinforce critical thinking skills, prioritization, data analysis methods, problem-solving, and nursing interventions. Games are specialty

Box 4–3.
Match Game

"Sunsetting" eyes, bulging fontanel	Increased intracranial pressure
Sunken fontanel, dry mucus membranes	Dehydration
No stools, can't pass rectal thermometer	Imperforate anus
Positive Barlow's and Ortolani's signs	Developmental hip dysplasia
Respiratory distress, formula from nose	Cleft palate
Tremors, lethargy	Hypoglycemia
Machine-like heart murmur	Patent ductus arteriosus
Small pustular rash	Milia
Cheeselike substance on skin	Vernix caseosa
Meatus under penis	Hypospadias

specific; I've used the pediatric edition in pediatric clinical post-conferences.

- A new game called "What Next?"[7] provides unfolding case studies that reflect complex, dynamic client conditions. These games are valuable in nursing orientation groups and classes on decision-making. For more information see Free[6,7] or www.whatifgame. homestead.com.

- Technology has greatly advanced our **Gaming** opportunities. There are many Web sites to assist with game construction and development. A word of caution: games take a lot of class time. Always keep class objectives in mind to ensure that **Gaming** stays on task.

- Paul and Elder[8] proposed a game entitled *Deck of Events.* Instructors use a deck of index cards, each with a critical thinking exercise or clinical question. The authors propose that instructors design their own clinical question deck and use these to challenge students during free time in the clinical area or at post-conference.

- If using **Gaming** as a test review, make a **Worksheet** of the major concepts and allow students to fill in the blanks. This technique allows the game to proceed in a more controlled fashion.

- Imitating the television show *What's My Line?,* Bowles[5] proposed forming panels of students who represent specific diseases, diagnoses, or procedures. Other students question the panel in order to guess their identities. Bowles also cites a game entitled *Reverse Bingo* as a means to review class material. The instructor prepares a bingo card for each student. Only one card has the answers to all 25 questions in the game. The instructor calls out the 25 questions, and students cover each answer as the matching question is asked. The winning student fills the bingo card and correctly answers the 25 questions.

Imagine and Remember When

General Description   Teaching empathy to new nurses can be a challenge. Asking students to **Imagine** living through an ordeal and using personal imagery to describe the emotions evoked is a valuable way to enhance sensitivity. Krejci[9] describes imagery as a means to let students develop mental models of learned material, and then practice it to master skills and acquire knowledge.

Remember When asks students to step back in time to remember a situation in their own lives similar to the one being discussed in class. Again, empathic understanding is the key lesson in this exercise.

Preparation and Equipment   There is little preparation for this exercise. Consider class content for which these strategies may be appropriate. You may want to create slides to formalize the exercise and encourage students to see its value.

Example of the Strategy at Work   In a class about children's responses to surgery and hospitalization, I used an imagery exercise slide to help my students **Imagine** (Box 4–4). We then discussed the developmental considerations of caring for pediatric clients, the fears children have in the clinical area, and the nurse's role in helping children cope with these stressors. I applied **Remember When** in a course on adolescent health behavior, asking students to think back to some of the struggles associated with the adolescent years (Box 4–5).

For many students, the illness, pain, and injury they witness in the clinical area are foreign to their personal experience. **Imagine** helps these students contemplate the impact such stressors would have on their personal lives.

In contrast, many students can draw on personal or familial events to develop or enhance empathy skills. **Remember When** allows students to share these personal experiences in class. For life skills classes, such as assertiveness, conflict resolution, or stress management, **Remember When** is a great way to uncover previous experiences and discuss how they were resolved. Coming up with alternative resolutions and discussing consequences will foster problem-solving skills.

Box 4–4.
Imagine

You are 6 years old. You've been admitted to the hospital after a tonsillectomy. You're having significant pain from the surgical site. Your mother is staying with you in the hospital. Your roommate is a 1-year-old with "a bad cold."

You don't want to express your pain because the nurse will make you swallow yucky medicine. The nurse tells your mom, with you listening, that you can't go home until you drink and pee. You don't like strange potties. It hurts to drink.

Now it's getting dark and you're afraid. Your mom has gone to the bathroom. The IV pump at your bedside starts to beep. People are talking in the hall, but you're lonely. You want to go home. You feel a tear fall down your cheek. You wipe it away and the IV board on your hand scratches you.

The nurse comes in and says hi, smiles, and turns on the bright lights. He's holding a drink, an electric thermometer, and a chart. You can tell he means business. Your mom isn't back yet, and you're really scared!

Ideas for Use

- Many people enter nursing because of personal experiences with health care or illness. **Remember When** provides a mechanism for catharsis and vicarious learning. You may need to guide this discussion if it gets off track or more detailed than class time will allow.
- **Imagine** may be used as a personal role-play exercise. Students build empathy by picturing what it would be like to experience any of the conditions discussed in class. Some **Imagine** exercises may be so realistic that they stimulate significant emotional responses. Instructors need to assess classes and provide debriefing or personal attention as needed.[10]
- Many athletes use **Imagine** or some

Box 4–5.
Remember When

Remember your adolescent years:
- Your level of self-esteem
- Your peer pressures
- Your parent's expectations
- Your own concerns and expectations
- Societal issues and pressures

other type of imagery to mentally accomplish a task, win a race, or reach a goal. Have your students **Imagine** changing a dressing, inserting a nasogastric tube, providing tracheostomy care, or administering an injection— they may master these skills more easily. Newer research is examining the value of **Imagine** for teaching psychomotor skills, approaches to care situations, and ways to handle unexpected circumstances.[8]

- Combine **Imagine** or **Remember When** with **Write to Learn** or **Quick Writes** to let students reflect on these exercises.
- In both strategies, ask students to focus on the emotions evoked during the scenarios. Have the class discuss these emotions and the role they play in fostering empathy. Ask the students to consider the client's reactions to the nonempathic nurse.
- One creative colleague assigns freshmen students the first *Harry Potter* novel, in which Harry arrives at his new school.[11] The instructor asks the class to **Imagine** their new life as college students. How are their experiences similar to Harry's? How are they different? What a great way to help new students examine their personal lives and emotions!
- Construct an **E-mail Exercise** asking students to **Remember When** and discuss a time when they confronted a challenge or obstacle. Ask them to compare and contrast this event with the challenge a client faces when receiving a new medical diagnosis.
- Foster relationships by asking practicing nurses to **Remember When** they were students or novice nurses.

Twosies

General description   In this strategy, students pair up to accomplish a task. This exercise may be very brief or more involved. Pairs can stay together for a single exercise or throughout the session or even longer. The small size of the group helps students get comfortable with the exercise. This strategy is less elaborate than **Think-Pair-Share.** In **Twosies,** students simply pair up for the exercise and complete the task.

Preparation and Equipment   Little preparation or equipment is needed, but you must plan when to use **Twosies** and how to make it work in class.

Example of the Strategy at Work   I have used this strategy in several ways. When discussing how nonverbal gestures and facial expressions affect communication, I ask the **Twosie** partners to say to each other, "I like your shirt," twice. The first time they use positive nonverbal signals: a pleasant tone and expression convey sincerity. The second time they frown and speak in a disdainful tone, their insincerity obvious. The students quickly get the importance of nonverbal communication and understand why a nurse must assess both verbal and nonverbal modes when "reading" a client. In addition, students are encouraged to consider their own nonverbal messages to which clients may be exposed. In the same class the students showed each other expressions of happiness, anger, sadness, and fear, reinforcing the role of facial expressions in communication and client assessment. I used **Twosies** again in a class on pain assessment, emphasizing the need to evaluate facial grimacing as a nonverbal sign of pain.

Students in my assessment class paired up and looked at each other's shoes. I asked them to come up with 10 words to describe those shoes—old, new, dirty, clean, big, little, what color, and so on. I pointed out that they'd just done an assessment. We discussed the words they would use and the things they would look for when assessing clients, families, and communities. Used this way, **Twosies** brings home the nature of assessment and the need for assessment skills in comprehensive care. Students realized the need to learn both the techniques and the terminology of assessment.

Brain teasers, games, and activities may be used in **Twosie** pairs. Here's a game I participated in at a conference. It's best done with students who are experienced travelers. You can use it as an icebreaker or as a **Twosie** to build rapport. Pairs work together to identify the following airport abbreviations. This is a stumper for even the most seasoned traveler. Answers follow, and some will surprise you.

Name that Airport

United States
1. LAS ＿＿＿
2. SMF ＿＿＿
3. RSW ＿＿＿
4. HNL ＿＿＿
5. LAX ＿＿＿
6. MCO ＿＿＿
7. AUS ＿＿＿
8. TPA ＿＿＿
9. JAX ＿＿＿
10. MSP ＿＿＿

International
11. HKG ＿＿＿
12. CDG ＿＿＿
13. ATH ＿＿＿
14. TXL ＿＿＿
15. PEK ＿＿＿
16. VCE ＿＿＿
17. YYZ ＿＿＿
18. SYD ＿＿＿
19. FCO ＿＿＿
20. SVO ＿＿＿

Answers	Answers
1. Las Vegas	11. Hong Kong
2. Sacramento	12. Paris
3. Fort Myers	13. Athens
4. Honolulu	14. Berlin
5. Los Angeles	15. Beijing
6. Orlando	16. Venice
7. Austin	17. Toronto
8. Tampa	18. Sydney
9. Jacksonville	19. Rome
10. Minneapolis	20. Moscow

Ideas for Use

- **Twosies** is an excellent strategy to use in large classes where students don't know each other or where group work may become too cumbersome.
- **Twosie** pairs can address any exercise, assignment, or question.
- Use tavern and children's puzzles, **Clinical Decision-making Exercises,** and other creative strategies to develop **Twosie** activities.
- **Twosie** exercises are great ways to learn technical clinical information. Have pairs work on interpreting ECG strips, deciphering lab results, interpreting blood gas values, calculating medication dosages, troubleshooting equipment, answering complex questions, or wading through the **Muddiest Part** of class content.

What's the Point? or What's the Big Deal?

General Description   This strategy is named after one of my personal experiences in nursing school. After making a grave but not life-threatening medication error, I said to my clinical instructor, "Well, what's the big deal?" That phrase has haunted me throughout my years as nurse and educator—I didn't know, but should have, what the big deal was. Now my role as nurse educator is to teach students **What's the Big Deal.**

Practicing nurses usually know what the priorities are and **What's the Big Deal**. Novices may need some guidance in discerning priorities, especially in complex situations. This strategy provides that guidance.

After presenting content or a client case, ask students, **What's the Point?** or **What's the Big Deal?** Grounding content and emphasizing priorities are vital not only in nursing care, but for passing the NCLEX-RN® examination.

Preparation and Equipment   Consider the right time to ask these questions in class. The timing depends on the level of your students, the course content, and the priorities you wish to emphasize. Priority setting requires subtle thinking and may be difficult at first—students must differentiate between intricate data sets to discover which priorities are highest. Experienced nurses may practice this skill intuitively, but new nurses and students benefit greatly from practice.

Example of the Strategy at Work   I use this strategy in many of the lectures I present. It's a great way to get attention. Sometimes, when the class is writing notes with heads bowed, I ask, **"What's the Big Deal?"** or **"What's the Point?"** It usually surprises me to see the heads pop up. Suddenly the students are all ears—they want to know the answers. They may just be curious. They may also realize that cue questions mean "This is important and may be on the test."

Simply asking these questions starts the "thinking machine" in students' minds. For example, in a pharmacology class we were discussing nitroglycerin and its actions in relieving angina. We discussed client education and the side effects of the medication. Sildenafil (Viagra) is contraindicated with nitroglycerine. By simply saying, **"What's the Big Deal?,"** I helped students realize that potentially life-threatening hypotension could result from an interaction. My question brought home the importance of this issue in clinical assessment.

In another class we were discussing sickle cell crisis and the significance of abdominal distention. I presented a **Quickie Case Study** in which the nurse notes that the client's blood pressure is lower than previous values. I asked, **"What's the Point?"** The class discussed the implications of abdominal distention and falling blood pressure: possible sequestration crisis, splenic rupture, and shock. When I placed the situation in this framework, the students understood its gravity.

In a seminar for seniors, we discussed their progress through nursing school and their ability to now "think like a nurse." In that discussion, we talked of the following client picture. Students were asked to consider what their concerns would have been freshman year as novices and now as graduating seniors. The scene: A 4-year-old client enters the ER with a high fever, nuchal rigidity, a decreased level of consciousness, and a rash on her entire torso—**What is the big deal?** To the novice student, a fever and rash do not seem serious. In contrast, experienced nurses know the signs of bacterial meningitis with potentially life-threatening outcomes and find this situation a grave one—needing immediate nursing and medical care.

Ideas for Use

- Use these questions any time you want to convey the seriousness of a condition or the importance of a nursing intervention. If you use them often, students will soon recognize these questions as a signal designating important information.

- These questions enhance test-taking skills. Here's a common student frustration with multiple-choice nursing examinations: often all four answers are correct. Students are expected to pick the *best* answer. This strategy helps them discriminate enough to choose the highest priority.

- Use **Case Studies** to set the climate for these questions. Have students sift through to find the most significant data by asking, **"What's the Big Deal?"**

- Use these questions to ask students to relate class content to their personal or clinical experiences.

- For a lesson in diversity, ask, **"What's the Point?"** when discussing cultural or spiritual priorities. Students are often surprised to discover the variety of their classmates' attitudes toward these issues. This strategy provides insight into the importance of assessing and respecting the cultural or spiritual aspects of a client's life.

Jigsaw

General Description   As the title suggests, this strategy is designed like a jigsaw puzzle. Each piece represents information that contributes to the whole picture but may not mean much in itself. Students learn that their piece of the puzzle—their contribution—is an important part of the whole; as systems theory tells us, the whole is greater than the sum of its parts. This strategy, first described by Aronson et al,[12] has been used extensively in nursing, education, and medicine to teach group problem-solving and course content.

Preparation and Equipment   In **Jigsaw** you need to break the class content or objectives into manageable chunks. These chunks represent the pieces of the puzzle, which can be completed by a group, pair, or individual. You then give each group the assignment and a time frame for the task. You also must allot time for sharing in the classroom, or come up with a way to communicate findings to all the students.

Example of the Strategy at Work   I used this exercise in a class on pediatric orthopedic anomalies. The class was designed to discuss five or six diagnoses. There were significant commonalities among the different conditions. I decided to form groups to work on each diagnosis so we could discuss these similarities in class, which included pain control, postsurgical care, neurovascular assessment, skin care, immobility, and developmental care.

In preparation for the class I assembled a list of conditions from the course objectives. They included developmental hip dysplasia, scoliosis, Legg-Calvé-Perthes disease, slipped capital femoral epiphysis, and talipes equinovarus (clubfoot). Each group was assigned a diagnosis. I asked the students to bring their pediatric text and be ready to work. To give each group its assignment I used a colorful slide (Fig. 4–2).

- For each disorder the group had the following responsibilities:
    - Define the disorder and the pathophysiology (identify organic changes).
    - Identify five to six assessments and diagnostic tests to detect and differentiate this disorder.

TODAY'S ACTIVITY
for each disorder:

- **Organic Changes** (Define the disorder and the pathophysiology)

- **Assessment** (Identify 5–6 assessments and diagnostic tests to detect/differentiate this disorder)

- **List 5–6 Management Strategies**

- **List 5–6 Nursing Considerations** (Consider nursing role with treatments)

Fig. 4–2.   Jigsaw exercise for a class on pediatric orthopedic abnormalities.

- List five to six management strategies.
- Identify five to six nursing considerations—consider the nurse's role in each treatment.

I printed out the slides I'd created for each diagnosis and gave each group the appropriate printout as a **Worksheet.** We then reconvened to discuss the exercise and the common components of care. Students discussed the surgical procedures, pain issues, assessments, and the role of the nurse in the care of these children. Students were encouraged to take notes on each other's presentations. The **Worksheets** were posted outside the classroom. Test questions were derived from the content of the **Worksheets** and from the notes.

Ideas for Use

- This strategy requires significant student "buy-in." The first time I used it, only two of more than a 100 students remembered to bring their text. As a result, the exercise was so devalued that I ended up delivering a traditional lecture. The next time this class came around I emphasized the students' need to bring their pediatric texts and assured them that test questions would be derived from the exercise.
- You may wish to do a smaller version of **Jigsaw** in a discussion group or clinical group (see **Clinical Puzzle**).
- Use **Case studies** to develop a **Jigsaw** exercise. In this exercise, it's necessary to show that each group member's contribution is integral to the whole.
- Make sure to set specific and realistic time limits so students use their time well.
- Circulate in the classroom to answer questions and keep the class on track.
- Post the **Worksheets** and the groups' conclusions on a bulletin board or on the Internet.
- Groups can give mini-seminars in class. Encourage students to take notes on their classmates' findings.
- Use **Jigsaw** as a way to teach project management, group process, and other exercises that foster teamwork.

Clinical Decision-making Exercises

General Description   **Clinical Decision-making Exercises** help students learn critical thinking and problem-solving skills. Resolution of conflicts and other problems is based on case studies and "interviews."

Each case study is developed to coincide with class content and objectives, and students apply the decision-making strategies they've discussed in class. In addition to these skills, they can draw on personal experience and clinical information.

Preparation and Equipment   You will need to develop the case study and questions in advance. Consider the decision-making strategies you've taught in class, and design cases to challenge the students' problem-solving skills.

Continuing education and staff development instructors can use a single case study for a needed break during class or in-services. It's an effective way to reinforce points of interest. Academic instructors will need to develop a grading system and explain it in the class syllabus. One downside of these assignments is that they can take a long time to correct and log in. What better opportunity to put teaching assistants or graduate students to work?

It's rewarding to read the students' answers, which generally demonstrate insight and thought. Here are the grading system and instructions I use with this assignment:

Students will read cases, interviews, and scenarios via WEB CT™. Students will answer questions and provide reflections via e-mail responses. E-mails must be sent to class teaching assistants via WEB CT. They are sent using the e-mail assignment/mailbox icon on the course home page. No e-mails are accepted if received via other e-mail routes.

Clinical decision making assignments are due by 5:00 PM on the date given in the class schedule. No assignments are accepted late!
Grading Rubric:

2 points: Submission meets assignment objectives, was on time.

1 point: Submission does not fully meet assignment objectives, was on time.

0 points: Submission was not on time, was not done, or did not meet assignment objectives.

Example of the Strategy at Work   Here are some of the assignments I used in an introductory nursing class. You can see how easily this assignment may be adapted for the content of your class.

Clinical Decision-making: Assignment 1

Hello. My name is Margaret Sanger. I am best known for my work in advocating for birth control to provide women with choices about their fertility. I am a nurse, but I found the occupation somewhat confining and decided to work as both a nurse and a socially conscious citizen.

Early in my career as a public health nurse, I saw women who were forced to bear many children because they lacked family planning resources and information. I was present at the death of a woman who had had several children in a few years, had no health care resources, and was financially unable to support her growing family. When I was taken to her third-floor apartment, I noted the dirty, poverty-ridden environment. The client later died of hemorrhage and infection. I vowed I would devote my life work to affording every woman the right to control conception.

I found that rich women had access to information and birth control methods from Europe. Poor women, who had an even greater reason to control conceptions, were lacking in such resources. My efforts in providing birth control information included writing documents about family planning, traveling to other countries to research their contraceptive practices, and lobbying for the provision of birth control to the public. I was scorned for my work, arrested in several states because of the information I had disseminated, and criticized for my stance on women's rights and choices.

At the time, women had just been granted the right to vote. Many legislators and other men in the United States still believed that entitlement to be wrong. Birth control was considered a private, "non-discussed" issues among many policy makers—who were, of course, male. Yet I challenge each of them to consider their own sexual practices. I challenge them also to think of their own children, and to consider childbearing and childrearing from the perspective of a woman. If they were not wearing the cloak of denial, they might feel very differently and might change their belief that birth control is only a woman's concern.

Many people accused me of wanting to control births among the poorer lower classes because I wanted to create a superior race. I must defend my efforts by saying that it is the poor who most direly need access to and information about birth control. I in no way wish to create another segment of society. In contrast, I want to let women enjoy sexual activity without the constant fear of pregnancy. I want to let families grow to their desired, affordable, and optimal size. I want to give women a way to function in the workforce and the public world in an arena of choice and autonomy.

These beliefs are rooted in my background as a nurse and in my philosophy about human rights. I do not regret the years I devoted to these initiatives. In fact, these early accomplishments led to the development of the Planned Parenthood Foundation, later known as the International Planned Parenthood Foundation. I hope these words provide insight into the decision-making that was once required of nurses, and the impact of those nurses on today's practice.

1. Cite one aspect of Margaret Sanger's life that exemplifies clinical decision-making.
2. Name one social, gender, or historical factor that may have influenced Margaret Sanger's efforts.
3. Name one way you might generalize the key points of this scenario to your own nursing values and practice in clinical decision-making.

Clinical Decision-making: Assignment 2

Hello. My name is John James. I am the nurse manager of an oncology unit at a major hospital center. I deal with many staff issues relating to professionalism and the image of nursing as a profession.

Nursing has given me the opportunity to practice nursing science independently and use my clinical decision-making skills every day. I work in collaboration with many other health professionals, but I feel self-directed and independent in my practice. Many people ask me why, as a man, I went into nursing. I'd always wanted to help people and provide a service to the community. I also felt that people look up to nurses for their knowledge. People who need care trust nurses.

When I got out of high school I wasn't sure what I wanted to do. I worked in a restaurant for a while. Then I had to have my appendix out. I watched the nurses and thought, "I can do that!" I decided to go to a university to get a BSN.

I belong to two nursing organizations: the American Nurses Association (ANA) and the Oncology Nursing Society. In these groups I can actively advocate for my clients. The ANA, for example, wrote the *Nursing Code of Ethics,* which guides me in providing safe, confident, and respectful care. I participate in nursing research. Our unit is studying pain management in cancer clients and is researching ways to help families with the grieving process.

Nursing research helps with the many questions I want answered. One problem I'd like to work on is the best way to take blood pressures. Nurses do that assessment all the time and don't realize how important it is. On my unit we've been discussing whether a blood pressure in the forearm will be the same as one in the upper arm. The results of that research may change my nursing assessments and the way I practice.

1. Cite five criteria of professionalism noted in this scenario.
2. Name one way in which these criteria can influence clinical decision-making.
3. Without looking at any research, describe in one sentence what you think about using the forearm instead of the upper arm to assess blood pressure.

Clinical Decision-making: Assignment 3

Mr. Truman was admitted to the hospital on November 1, after experiencing chest pain and shortness of breath. He had undergone cardiac surgery about 10 years before and was beginning to have symptoms again. He was scheduled for a cardiac catheterization, but it was delayed until November 3 because of technical problems. The physician also referred Mr. Truman to a diet counselor for a low-cholesterol diet.

The cardiac catheterization was done without complications and no surgery was indicated. Mr. Truman was hospitalized overnight for observation. On November 4, it was noted that he had a low-grade fever. He was treated with acetaminophen and given three doses of IV antibiotics. His temperature returned to normal and he was discharged on November 5.

Principal diagnosis: Ischemia, heart disease
Secondary diagnosis: Disturbances heart, functional—long-term effect of cardiac surgery
Diagnosis-related group assigned: DRG 125: circulatory disorders except acute myocardial infarction with cardiac catheterization without complex diagnosis.
Allowed length of stay: 2.2 days
Actual length of stay: 4.1 days
DRG Payment per discharge = $6800.00

Actual hospital costs = $10, 348.00
Loss for hospital = $3548.00

1. How did the technical problems and Mr. Truman's temperature affect the length of his hospital stay and the hospital costs?
2. How can a hospital make up the lost funds?
3. State one impact of health-care financing on clinical decision-making.

Clinical Decision-making: Assignment 4

Hello. My name is Joe Jones. I am 38 years old. About 10 years ago, I was a wild guy. I was drinking and riding a motorcycle without a helmet. I hit a wet spot in the road and slid. My bike went out from under me and I fell head first into the road. Witnesses said I took a dive into the ground.

After the accident I was unable to move anything from the waist down. I was taken by helicopter to a trauma center, put on a ventilator, and supported through IV fluids and nutrition. I was eventually able to breathe on my own and eat real food. I spent 3 months in a hospital rehabilitation unit learning to take care of myself. I learned how to do my own activities of daily living, live within my environment, and relate to others with my new abilities and disabilities. I've become quite independent.

Nurses took care of me in the period right after my injury, monitoring vital signs, assessing my status, and providing lots of physical care. As I progressed, nurses helped me learn how to lead a fulfilling life. I am married, we have one child, and I work at a library. I'm sad that I can't walk, but in many ways my life is better because of my life-changing accident.

1. After reviewing Neuman's Systems Theory or the School of Nursing Organizational Framework, state how each defines each component of the metaparadigm: nurse, client, environment, and health.
2. State one way in which either theory can influence clinical decision-making.
3. After reading the scenario, state two ways in which the either theory may be used to interpret this situation.

Clinical Decision-making: Assignment 5

I'll tell you a story from when I was a new nurse. On my first week-end as an RN, I was in the middle of admitting a client who had sustained a hip fracture. The client was 75 years old and had fallen while going to the bathroom. In my opinion, a person that old should be in a nursing home anyway.

So, the client fell and I was assigned to take care of him. I knew he was alert and oriented, but I would have felt better getting a history from someone who wasn't so old and feeble. I finished the admission, and traction was ordered for the client. As a new nurse, I wasn't skilled at doing traction. I never learned how to set up traction in school or in hospital orientation, but I decided to do my best.

I put the client in traction and moved on to my other clients. The client complained of pain about 1 hour later, and I gave him a shot of analgesic in the right buttock. He jumped a little at the injection, but later expressed pain relief. I checked the traction and took the vital signs; everything appeared to be fine. I moved on to care for my other six clients.

About 4 hours later, the client again complained of pain. I prepared and administered the pain medication in the left buttock. The client exclaimed that he didn't even feel the injection. I thought, "I must be getting better!" I checked the traction and moved on to my other duties. Then I reported to the next shift and left for the day.

When I returned the next day, I found to my surprise that all was not well. The traction had been improperly applied, and the client had suffered permanent nerve damage. The client required surgery, sustained tissue destruction, and was very angry with his nursing care. I felt frustrated—after all, I'd done the best I could. These old folks can be so unreasonable! I felt angry with nursing, my agency, and this client. What else could I have done?

1. Name one legal principle violated in this scenario.
2. Name one ethical principle violated in this scenario.
3. Name one way these violations may affect clinical decision-making.
4. Using sound clinical decision-making skills, state what else could have been done.

Clinical Decision-making: Assignment 6

Use Lewin's theory of change to reflect on clinical decision-making skills. How do the concepts of unfreezing, moving, and refreezing relate to your personal development of clinical decision-making skills throughout the semester?

Clinical Decision-making: Assignment 7

After your field experience, answer the following questions:

1. How did you prepare for this experience?
2. State the values of any screening results not within normal limits. Use your clinical decision-making skills.
3. What recommendations did you make, or could you have made, based on these values?

Ideas for Use

- Use **Clinical Decision-making Exercises** to evaluate understanding of class content. Reinforce concepts as needed. If assignments are done weekly or bi-weekly, you can routinely assess the students' understanding and need for additional practice.
- Have students document **Clinical Decision-making Exercises** in an **Ah-hah Journal** and hand it in at the end of the semester or rotation.
- For new nurses, use a **Clinical Decision-making Exercise** each day of nursing orientation. This reinforces critical thinking skills and helps staff get to know the clients most commonly cared for in their clinical environment.
- Students can complete **Clinical Decision-making Exercises** in pairs or trios as part of a classroom activity.
- Students may write these exercises, post them in an **Online Discussion**, or send them as an **E-mail Exercise.**
- Make sure that class examinations reflect the concepts discussed in **Clinical Decision-making Exercises.**
- Consider peer grading: have students evaluate each other's exercises using instructor-developed criteria.
- Nursing specialty classes and specialty unit orientations are rich in nursing decisions. Use **Clinical Decision-making Exercises** as an entertaining way to review class content.

Reality Check

General Description   The words **Reality Check** can frame a theoretical discussion in the context of real nursing practice. Clinical examples provide a mechanism for discussion. This strategy is an excellent way for students to differentiate between real-life health-care issues and those they see on television and read about in fiction.

In **Reality Check,** material is introduced theoretically and then given a real context. The instructor centers class topics on actual evidence and true events. **Reality Check** may be based on real clinical cases (with names omitted). Physical evidence can include hospital bills, replications of clinical records, or simulated charting. Just by saying **"Reality Check,"** you'll prompt your students to consider some of the issues that affect health care and their role in safe nursing practice.

Preparation and Equipment   Use your clinical practice affiliations to obtain real hospital costs, documentation samples, and other evidence (Fig. 4–3). This exercise is a great opportunity to discuss the financial side of health care and demonstrate the burden it places on individuals, industry, and public resources.

Example of the Strategy at Work   I use a slide on the idea of Figure 4–3 as a **Reality Check** in a pharmacology class. It is easy for us to just say "medications cost a lot." Instead, we can provide physical evidence of these costs from a real client experience to drive home these points.

After viewing the slide, we discuss the impact of health-care costs on someone without insurance or adequate financial resources. Seeing the physical evidence brings home the reality to students. The fiscal aspects of nursing and health care are a key part of the **Reality Check** nurses need to practice responsibly and safely.

Ideas for Use

- Instead of using physical evidence, just say **"Reality Check"** when it's time to think about putting a theory into action. You can use some questions to stimulate discussions:
  - How does this information relate to the real world?
  - How often does a nurse have time to sit down and talk with a client the way we just discussed?
  - How does a nurse care for such an ill client along with several other clients?
  - How does a nurse juggle several priorities at once?
- This strategy can highlight legal and ethical issues. It can also illustrate the workforce issues associated with nursing, such as nurse-to-client ratios, delegation, unionization, pulling (sending

REALITY CHECK

CPT:	99211 OV LEVEL 1	36.00
CPT:	90780 IV THERAPY 1ST HR	118.00
CPT:	J1642 HEPARIN FLUSH, PER 10 UNITS	4.00
CPT:	96530 REFILL/MAINT INPLANT PUMP	68.00
CPT:	J7030 1000CC NORMAL SALINE	22.50
CPT:	J7050 NORMAL SALINE 250 ML	22.50
CPT:	96410 CHEMO INF TO 1 HR	198.00
CPT:	96410ST TRAY FEE	75.00
CPT:	J9214 INTERFERON ALFA, 1 MIL	746.24

This is the cost/treatment. Treatments are 5x/week for 12 months: 1300 x 5 x 52 = **$338,000.00!!!!!** Does not include lab work, other medications, other health visits, transportation to treatments, other health concerns, durable medical supplies, nutritional supplements, diagnostics, radiation/chemo/surgery expenses, etc.

nurses to other units), cross-training (orienting nursing staff to multiple specialties), and professional issues.

- Hunt[13] provides a great resource for making client care more realistic. This **Reality Check** exercise is called "Armchair Shopper." Clients are given a list of questions and asked for solutions. I'm sure you'll agree that these questions, inspired by the "Armchair Shopper," are also great **Reality Checks** for new nurses and nursing students:
  - How would you navigate your snowy yard in a wheelchair?
  - How would you plan your daily diet to keep your sodium restricted?
  - How would you change your father's diaper in a public restroom?
  - How would you transfer your mother, with right-sided hemiplegia, into and out of the passenger side of the car?
  - Looking at this restaurant menu, what selections would you make to adhere to your prescribed diet?

- You medication must be kept cold at all times. How would your transport it on vacation?
- What would you do if you dropped or broke your last vial of insulin on the ground on a weekend?
- What would you do if a client suffered a cardiac arrest on an elevator and you were the only person there?
- How would you respond if a client said he was leaving the hospital even though he had not been discharged?
- What resources would you need to change a dressing for a client you were caring for?
- What would you do if an IV bag ran dry and there were no other bags of that solution on the floor?

You can adapt the questions, as I have here, for inpatient care or keep them home-based for client education.

Muddiest Part

General Description   This strategy was shared with me at a class I taught about creative teaching strategies. After some research, I discovered that **Muddiest Part** was developed by Mosteller[14] as a means to assess class learning. The original strategy was called "Muddiest Point." The term denotes the part of a class that students, instructors, or both consider the most confusing or complex.

In nursing education, we can often tell when we've reached the **Muddiest Part.** Students shake their heads or look frustrated. You may hear a murmur in the crowd or see students craning their necks to find out whether their neighbor understood something better than they did. These are sure signs that you've reached a **Muddiest Part.** The next step is to clarify the material. You can do this either through class discussion or by using another creative teaching strategy to present the topic differently.

Preparation and Equipment   The only preparation needed is a sensitivity to the **Muddiest Parts** of a prepared class. Usually instructors can predict them and can build in additional time or plan a teaching strategy to allay fears. Sometimes, however, students may encounter a **Muddiest Part** when the instructor least expects it. Teachers need to be vigilant for signs of frustration and confusion.

Example of the Strategy at Work   It's a good idea to peruse your lecture material and try to determine the **Muddiest Parts.** You can trudge through the mud in advance by planning a creative strategy to reinforce material. Most experienced nurses and nurse educators remember the usual areas of confusion: the neuroendocrine system, ventilator settings, interpreting arterial blood gases, calculating vasopressor drips, using chest tubes to treat a pneumothorax . . . the list is endless.

When you see a wave of mud break over the class, step back and clarify. Provide additional information or suggest additional resources to clear up the confusion. To assess the **Muddiest Part** by watching the class, I look for both verbal and nonverbal cues when discussing complex information.

Ideas for Use

- Students often feel relieved when they realize that a **Muddiest Part** also confuses other people.
- Ask students to identify the **Muddiest Part** in a class as an assessment technique. Use **Admit Tickets** or Exit Tickets , **E-mail Exercises, Ah-hah Journals,** or **Online Discussion Groups** to collect these responses. Provide support in subsequent classes by contributing to **Online Discussion Groups,** posting information to Web-based bulletin boards, or using other innovative strategies.
- If you teach the same content repeatedly, use **Muddiest Parts** to provide insight for future teaching experiences.

In-class Test Questions

General Description   Nursing students, especially seniors gearing up for NCLEX-RN®, are very responsive to test questions scattered throughout a lecture. New nurses in orientation groups benefit from intermittent testing of skills. Experienced nurses—especially those taking objective examinations for certification or course completion—appreciate revisiting multiple-choice test items. What better way to brush up on test-taking skills? In this strategy, the instructor inserts appropriate test questions in the lecture. **In-class Test Questions** help you assess the class, help the class determine what they know, and provide an opportunity to practice testing skills.

Preparation and Equipment   All you need to do is develop test questions based on the lecture or discussion material. Questions may be placed in PowerPoint format. Animation may be added—for example, you can use an arrow to pinpoint, enlarge, or highlight the correct answer. It's important to remove the arrows, or anything else that gives away the correct answer, before providing handouts. The students aren't supposed to have the answers in their notes! Present a question every 15 minutes or so to coincide with a learner's usual attention span.

Example of the Strategy at Work   This strategy is one of the most common ones I use for brief diversions during class. **In-class Test Questions** also provide transition points to new topics of discussion. Box 4–6 shows a sample question I use to demonstrate the strategy to groups of nurse educators.

In-class Test Questions are a great way to reinforce material and provide breaks in a lecture or discussion. This strategy comes with some cautions:

- Make sure the **In-class Test Questions** match the difficulty level of the examination questions. Students will feel overconfident and be misled if the questions are too easy. Overly difficult questions will frustrate and intimidate them.
- Use questions from previous examinations to show the students what your testing style is like and what level of difficulty to expect.
- Use as many application and analysis questions as possible. You'll be asking students to make a leap from simple retention to actual use of their knowledge. For example, here is a retention question:

Which of the following is a common complication after a splenectomy?

1. Infection
2. Venous thrombosis
3. **Pneumonia**
4. Dehydration

Box 4–6.
In-class Test Question

Active learning is effective for young people because:
1. They are all hyperactive and have short attention spans.
2. They suffer the effects of immobility, such as pressure areas on bony prominences,
3. They have the same learning styles.
4. **They learn best when participating in the teaching-learning process.**

The first question asks students to recall the most common complication of splenectomy: pneumonia caused by the location of the incision and the resulting postoperative pain, which limits the depth of respirations. Now it's time to leap from retention to application. Ask the students how to assess for that complication or prevent it. See the subtle differences in this question:

Which of the following nursing interventions would prevent the most common complication following a splenectomy?

1. Antibiotic therapy and wound cultures
2. Leg exercises and pneumatic compression boots
3. **Coughing and deep breathing exercises**
4. IV hydration and oral fluids

You can even take that questions one step further, asking the students to evaluate the effectiveness of the intervention, as in this question:

A client you are caring for is 1 day post-splenectomy. Which of the following assessments would indicate that interventions to prevent the most common complication of this surgery were effective?

1. Client is afebrile and incision is dry and intact
2. Negative Homans' sign and lack of extremity pain
3. **Clear breath sounds and normal work of breathing**
4. Good skin turgor and adequate urine output

For this question, students must first determine the complication and then identify the prevention strategy. Although antibiotics may be used to treat the pneumonia, a better answer is to prevent it with pulmonary hygiene.

- Adhere to the standards of test construction. Don't include personal names in questions. Limit the length of questions and cases to necessary information. Don't ask all-of-the-above or none-of-the-above questions. Make sure answers are correct and similar in format and length. Distribute correct answers evenly among the four letters or numbers. Make sure the questions adequately represent testable material. Newer guidelines suggest using the word "patient" rather than "client."
- When showing a test question in class, ask students to read it quietly and await your signal to call out the response. Nothing is more frustrating for slower readers than to have someone call out an answer before they've even finished reading the question and the answer choices.

Ideas for Use

- Have students develop their own test questions. Composing questions is a great way to study and brings home the difficulty of test construction. Use a **Twosies** exercise—have students develop questions and switch with their partners. Ask the class to post their questions to an **Online Discussion.**

Alternatively, have students hand in questions as **Admit Tickets** and tell them you might use their questions on the examination. You'll be giving the class a way to prepare and to participate in evaluation. These questions may also be useful for test review and study sessions. Encourage students to use them in study groups (see **Learning from Each Other**). Experience has taught me that students develop hard test questions! You may need to revise them for the examination.

- During **Student-led Seminars,** have students compose test questions and write them on an index card. You can ask these questions after the seminar to evaluate class participation and attentiveness. Again, you may find yourself selecting questions to use on an examination.

- Have students post their questions and answers with rationales to an **Online Discussion.** Not only can you use the questions for test development, but students can use them to study for the examination. A colleague provides extra credit to students whose questions were actually used for the examination.

- Hand out electronic clickers (or ask students to purchase them) to use in answering questions. Clickers are also good for taking attendance, conducting quizzes, and assessing knowledge. Personal response systems or "clickers" allow students to answer questions in PowerPoint and provide the instructor with some assessment of the class's level of comprehension.

- **In-class Test Questions** can come from textbooks, test banks, and nursing examination review books.

- Give the class a solid foundation for the NCLEX® examination. One student told me about "NCLEX World," where nurses have endless amounts of time, money, and resources to accomplish their tasks. This concept helps students select the correct action without considering constraints. Of course, in real clinical practice, resources are finite and nurses must often make some changes in their nursing care, still staying within the basic parameters of client safety, benefit, and respect.

- Nursing examinations typically offer four correct answers. Students often find it frustrating to have to select the best, first, or highest nursing priority. **In-class Test Questions** help them practice these skills in the classroom.

- When using **In-class Test Questions,** make sure you cover the correct answer with rationales and discuss the reasons the others are incorrect. Students often find review of the incorrect answers a great learning experience.

- Encourage the question "What do you think they'll ask about this topic on the examination?" Students often have a difficult time anticipating and differentiating priorities. Using questions on a regular basis will foster those skills.

- Give your students a test blueprint or guide. If they know the number of questions per topic, class objective, or hour of class, they can study according to those parameters.

- One seasoned nursing instructor recommends posting a test question on the board during a class break. Whether written, on an overhead slide, or in PowerPoint, the questions are reviewed when the class reconvenes. Because these questions may, or may not, appear on an examination, students are encouraged to return from the class break promptly.

- For more information on test construction and administration, see Oermann and Gaberson.[15]

E-mail Exercises

General Description   This strategy is effective in assessing knowledge level and in helping students keep up with class information. It's also a convenient way to distribute **Quick Write** or **Write to Learn** exercises. In **E-mail Exercises,** students e-mail the instructor or teaching assistants with brief assignments or answers to questions.

Preparation and Equipment   You'll need to compose the **E-mail Exercises** and establish both an evaluation mechanism and a policy regarding these assignments. Guidelines should be set out in the course syllabus.

Example of the Strategy at Work   I used **E-mail Exercises** throughout a pharmacology course as a key teaching and assessment strategy.

Here are the syllabus guidelines for **E-mail Exercises:**

E-mail Assignments

Eleven e-mail assignments are scheduled throughout the semester. See class schedules for the directions. Each e-mail must be received by 5:00 P.M. on the due date. A maximum of 10 points is available; one extra assignment is included to provide flexibility when needed. Assignments received by the due date and time will receive one point; assignments received late or not at all will receive zero points. E-mail exercises make up 10 percent of the grade in this course.

Exercise 1

You are asked to participate in a double-blind research study. All clients will be asked to take daily medication to treat their severe, uncomfortable, chronic disease. Half of the sample will be randomly designated to receive a medication with an excellent chance of curing the illness. The other half will be assigned to a control group and will receive a placebo.

This experimental treatment is the only one known for the illness. There is an informed consent procedure, and identities will be kept confidential. The subjects will receive $1000 to participate in the study for 6 months.

State two ways in which the principle of autonomy is respected in this study. State two ways in which autonomy is threatened.

Exercise 2

A client is to be discharged with a prescription for 10 mg of oral morphine. The oral morphine is available in a solution of 2 mg/mL. Calculate how much morphine the client should receive. While in the hospital he was receiving 3 mg of morphine by IV.

In two to three sentences, explain to the client why the oral dose is higher than the parenteral dose. Use your knowledge from the last few weeks to build your answer.

Exercise 3

A client with seizures is admitted to the hospital. He routinely takes phenytoin (Dilantin) as an anticonvulsant. His seizures were controlled until last night, when he had a grand mal seizure at home. His blood levels were drawn, and phenytoin was found to be below therapeutic level. His previous dose was 50 mg with breakfast and dinner and 75 mg at bedtime. Answer the following questions:

1. What could be the reason for the client's breakthrough seizures?
2. Is this client's dose of phenytoin appropriate?
3. Why is the monitoring of blood levels important?
4. Why is the bedtime dose greater than the other two doses?

Exercise 4

A 2-year-old girl visits the nurse practitioner. She is irritable, febrile, and has some nasal congestion. Her parents report that she is rubbing her ears and appears to be very uncomfortable. On the basis of physical examination and history, the nurse practitioner gives a diagnosis of otitis media and prescribes 125 mg of amoxicillin three times daily for 10 days. The amoxicillin suspension is available in 250 mg/5 mL.

1. How much medication should the child receive?
2. How often?
3. The mother asks if she can use household teaspoons. What is your response?
4. The father asks if the child needs to take the medicine for the entire 10 days if she starts to feel better. In two to three sentences, respond to his question.

Exercise 5

You are a home care nurse treating an elderly man who lives alone and whose purified protein derivative test and chest x-ray were positive for tuberculosis. He is being treated with three different antitubercular medications: isoniazid, ethambutol, and streptomycin. He asks why he can't take just one medication.

1. In two or three sentences, explain why multidrug therapy is indicated.
2. He has orders to have his blood drawn in 2 months for liver enzyme levels. Why?
3. After 3 months of therapy, he complains of ringing in his ears. What condition does this indicate and which medication could be responsible?

Exercise 6

A client has a diagnosis of leukemia. He complains of fatigue, shortness of breath, and weakness. The physician believes these symptoms are caused by anemia. The client is ordered to receive erythropoietin subcutaneously. In two to three sentences, describe the action of this medication. In two to three sentences, describe how to give a subcutaneous injection.

Exercise 7

A 52-year-old man is recovering from a heart attack. You are caring for him on a medical-surgical unit. He is ordered to receive digoxin.

1. What nursing precautions are essential during administration of this medication?
2. As a nurse, you are vigilant for signs and symptoms of digoxin toxicity. List several of these signs and symptoms.
3. You are aware that low levels of one electrolyte can potentiate (add to) digoxin toxicity. What is the electrolyte?

Exercise 8

A 16-year-old client with cystic fibrosis is ordered to receive fat-soluble vitamins in a water-soluble form. In two to three sentences, explain the difference between fat- and water-soluble vitamins. In one sentence, explain why this client should not take fat-soluble vitamins.

Exercise 9

A client is ordered to receive sucralfate (Carafate) for treatment of a peptic ulcer. Explain how this medication should be administered in relation to other medications and meals. Provide rationales for your answers.

Exercise 10

A client receives regular insulin at 7 a.m. At 10 a.m. he becomes shaky, irritable, and sweaty. Answer the following questions:

1. What do these symptoms indicate?
2. What characteristic of regular insulin predisposes to this problem?
3. What actions should the nurse take?

Exercise 11

A 22-year-old woman enters the gynecology clinic seeking oral contraception. Answer the following questions:

1. The client asks about the side effects of oral contraception. Summarize these.
2 The client smokes. What would you tell her?
3. The client reports taking St. John's Wort for depression.

What would you tell her?

As you can see, **E-mail Exercises** help students apply classroom principles, use problem-solving skills, and prepare for class. Key to this process is that e-mail exercises are assigned prior to coverage in class. This ensures a level of preparation for class such that class can proceed in a more effective manner.

Ideas for Use

- Checking and grading **E-mail Exercises** can be time-consuming and laborious, especially in a larger class. Teaching assistants or graduate students can help with grading.
- Use textbook exercises, **Clinical Decision-making Exercises,** or **Critical Thinking Exercises** as questions for this strategy.
- Make sure the exercises apply to current classes so students will have to prepare. Some of my students have said they'd prefer to have the **E-mail Exercises** follow a class discussion. I had to remind them that one purpose of this assignment is to encourage preparation before class.
- **E-mail Exercises** may be posted to **Online Discussion Groups** or to an electronic bulletin board.

Group Tests

General Description   In this effective strategy, students take a short test as a group. They're directed to answer the questions following a group discussion, in which all members reach a consensus about the correct answers. One of the most valuable parts of this strategy is the analysis of incorrect answers. The instructor leads with the question "Why are the other options incorrect?"

This strategy builds test-taking ability, fosters teamwork, encourages study groups, and helps the instructor assess the knowledge level of the class. Students learn valuable test-taking strategies from each other during group work.

Preparation and Equipment   You will need to develop a group test of five to 15 items, set aside class time, and establish the groups. (See **Group Thought** for some hints on the formation and use of group exercises.) The group at large can discuss the correct answers, you can grade the **Group Tests** and discuss them in class later, or correct answers with rationales may be posted in an **Online Discussion Group.**

Example of the Strategy at Work   This strategy has proved effective in a senior-level seminar course, a portion of which was devoted to NCLEX® preparation. Group tests were well received and gave the students a different way to practice test-taking strategies.

Here are two of my group tests:

Group Test 1   General Nursing Review

1. A nurse is ordered to administer 8500 units of heparin to a client by IV. The medication comes in 10,000 unit/mL concentration in 10-mL syringes. How many mL should the nurse administer?

   Answer: 0.85 mL

2. A client is crying as she approaches the nurses' station. The client yells at the nurse seated at the desk and says that she needs to see the Nurse Manager, slamming her fist down on the counter. The nurse correctly manages this client by

   a. Setting clear limits on the client's behaviors.
   b. Saying to the client "You seem upset."
   c. Ignoring the client's behavior.
   d. Referring the client to the nurse manager.

3. A client with diabetes mellitus is admitted to the unit with a history of alternating high and low sugar levels, poor compliance, and alcohol ingestion. The nurse enters the room and the client is unconscious but is breathing with a strong pulse. The nurse should

   a. Call the physician immediately.
   b. Check the client's blood sugar.
   c. Administer a STAT dose of insulin.
   d. Establish an IV line for dextrose injection.

4. The nurse is changing the dressing on a central venous catheter. Put the following steps in correct order:

   a. Assess the site.
   b. Don sterile gloves.
   c. Clean the site with antiseptic swabs.

d. Apply the clear transparent dressing.

e. Don clean gloves.

f. Remove the old dressing.

Order: E, F, A, B, C, D

5. A client has a nasogastric (NG) tube for decompression. The nurse irrigates the NG every 4 hours with 20 mL of normal saline solution. When doing the 8-hour shift totals, the nurse empties 260 mL of fluid from the drainage container. Calculate the true NG drainage for the shift.

Answer: 220 mL

Group Test 2   Management of Care and Delegation

1. An RN from the maternity unit is reassigned to the Emergency Department. Which of the following clients would be most appropriate to assign to this RN?

   a. A 50-year-old with chest pain and an ECG showing elevated ST segments

   b. A 25-year-old who fell from a ladder and has a fractured arm and no other trauma

   c. An elderly client in acute respiratory distress for whom the family wants "everything to be done"

   d. A 7-year-old with expiratory wheezing

2. Which client should the day shift RN assess immediately after receiving report from the night shift?

   a. A 76-year-old man with deep vein thrombosis being converted from IV heparin to oral warfarin

   b. A 45-year-old client with type 1 diabetes mellitus with a fasting blood glucose level of 130 who is hungry

   c. A 60-year-old client who had a tracheostomy placed yesterday and has a humidity collar

   d. A 75-year-old who had a transurethral prostatectomy 2 days ago and has a 3-lumen catheter

3. A client is to receive a feeding through an NG tube. Which task related to this activity could the RN delegate to the UAP?

   a. Checking the placement of the tube

   b. Documenting the feeding

   c. Flushing the tube with water before and after the feeding

   d. Accessing the formula from the nutrition department

4. Which client could the RN safely assign to the LPN to care for?

   a. A 70-year-old with a pulmonary embolus
   b. A 69-year-old with Prinzmetal's angina
   c. A 70-year-old who had a total hip replacement 3 days ago
   d. A 78-year-old receiving chemotherapy for breast cancer

5. An RN is assigned to admit a new client to a medical-surgical unit. The UAP can be delegated all of the following tasks except

   a. Escorting the client to her room
   b. Orienting the client to the bed and call bell system
   c. Helping the client change into a hospital gown
   d. Interviewing the client about medications and health history

6. An RN from a medical-surgical unit is pulled to the intensive care unit. Which of the following is appropriate to assign to the RN?

   a. A client awaiting transfer to the step-down unit
   b. A client in cardiogenic shock
   c. A client who has a pulmonary capillary wedge pressure monitor
   d. A client who has recently undergone open-heart surgery

7. An RN arrives for work and finds the shift very short-staffed. When the RN receives her client assignment, she feels she has been assigned too many clients to provide safe care for all of them. The nurse should report this problem to

   a. The nursing supervisor
   b. The charge nurse
   c. The unit clerk
   d. The director of nursing

8. A pediatric client is admitted with a new diagnosis of Wilms' tumor. The nurse is teaching the UAP key components of the client's care. The most important part of care is to:

   a. Assess for hematuria
   b. Frequently rate the client's abdominal pain
   c. Monitor urine output
   d. Refrain from palpation of the abdomen

9. A nurse is caring for a client who had major spinal surgery 8 hours ago. The nurse notes that the client has an NG tube to straight drainage, a peripheral IV, and a back dressing that is dry and intact.

The belly is distended and the client complains of mild abdominal pain. The nurse should

a. Empty the NG drainage container
b. Irrigate the NG tube
c. Assess bowel sounds
d. Provide an oral feeding

10. A client with ascites is scheduled for a paracentesis. The nurse is preparing the client for the procedure. Which of the following actions should be carried out initially?

a. Scrub the skin
b. Place the client in a high Fowler's position
c. Measure the client's abdominal girth
d. Check that the consent form is signed

11. A client is displaying all of the following lab work. Which of the following warrants the greatest concern?

a. A BUN of 25
b. A serum sodium of 140
c. A hematocrit of 45%
d. A white blood cell count of 500

12. An unknown relative brings a 6-year-old client to the Emergency Department. The client appears to need surgery. The first action of the nurse is to:

a. Prepare the client for surgery
b. Determine who may sign the surgical consent for the child
c. Teach the client about the operating room procedure
d. Access insurance information

Ideas for Use

- Using **Group Tests** early in a course allows the students to assess your testing style.
- Provide a **Group Test** as a review before examinations.
- Encourage students to work rapidly to foster test-taking skills. Even though NCLEX® and many certification examinations aren't strictly timed, they do have a maximum time limit.
- **Group Tests** are a great way to introduce students to some features of NCLEX® alternative items, question format, blueprints, level of difficulty, and priority setting.

- Make up groups with varying knowledge levels so students can model behavior and learn from each other.
- Use test banks or review books to construct **Group Tests.**
- **Group Tests** may be used in continuing education and in-services. Prizes and incentives make them more fun and increase the competition between groups.
- Administer **Group Tests** to pairs, trios, or larger groups. Encourage students to study together in the same groups.
- **Group Tests** may be constructed for any subject matter. To calculate the time needed for this exercise, allow about 1 minute per question and several minutes for discussion. It takes time to consider all answer options, but the time is well worth taking.

Web Assignments

General Description   The Internet has opened up a whole new way to access knowledge. We have an unprecedented amount of information at our fingertips. In **Web Assignments,** students are instructed to search the Internet for answers to assigned questions. Students either discuss their findings informally in class or send their insights as an **E-mail Exercise** or to an **Online Discussion Group.** Students can also e-mail the URL to the instructor for reference.

This strategy promotes awareness of online resources, both for health professionals and for the public. It also develops critiquing skills—students must make sure their information comes from a valid source.

Preparation and Equipment   The only preparation you need for this exercise is to search for Internet resources that students will find valuable.

Example of the Strategy at Work   I asked students in a health promotion class to search for smoking cessation Web sites. Part of the assignment was to print out the exercise or the home page and bring it in for discussion. This paper served as the **Admit Ticket** for the class. I showed a slide from the Centers for Disease Control and Prevention page on smoking cessation strategies. We began by discussing its value as a resource and moved on to cover some of the other sites the students had found.

I've also asked students to use a search engine to determine the number of Web sites available for selected topics. My students were surprised to find 65,000 Web site "hits" on diabetes and 33,000 on digoxin. It's important for nurses, especially when providing client education, to appreciate the sheer number of sites available to the public.

Ideas for Use

- Although most students know how to use the Internet these days, some are reluctant to enter this realm. **Web Assignments** help them practice the skills they need to search for health-related information.
- Devote some discussion time to providing criteria for your students to use in evaluating Web sites. This guidance will enhance their scholarly writing as well as their nursing practice.
- If your classroom has an Internet connection (wired or wireless), conduct a sample search in class using different search engines. Compare results and evaluate the selected Web sites.
- Have students **Think-Pair-Share** about their findings.
- Pose a question and ask students to search out the answer. They'll access an interesting variety of Web sites and, at times, provide a diversity of answers. Use this opportunity to discuss the reputability of the Internet as an information source.
- For a more extensive class project, have students develop a resource booklet of Web sites for specific client conditions.
- Use **Web Assignments** to create an in-service that introduces nursing staff to different electronic resources. Teach them to use the intranet within an organization, the agency's Internet resources; client education materials; and Internet resources approved for client distribution. To provide good education, nurses must know what information is available to clients and how valid the sources are.
- Ask students to critique a Web site, analyzing the validity of the source. Have them consider the ease of navigating the site—how difficult would it be for someone with less developed computer skills?
- Spend some time discussing the validity of online resources. This is a key skill for nursing professionals.

Student-led Seminars

General Description   In nursing education, **Student-led Seminars** are commonly used for clinical, agency, and discussion groups. This strategy provides a forum for practicing presentation and developing organizational skills. It also provides a teaching voice besides that of the instructor.

However, you need to observe some cautions. In its abbreviated, "on the run" form, the strategy requires a 10-minute time limit for the presentation. Students must differentiate "need-to-know" from "nice-to-know" and focus on information that takes priority. **Student-led Seminars** could become monotonous if you let them drag on. Besides focusing on priorities, this method encourages creativity and reinforces the premise of this book—that learning can be fun!

Preparation and Equipment   Develop a list of potential presentation topics and provide guidelines. These should include the information to be covered, the time frame, possible use of resources, research, stipulations for Internet use, and specific recommendations. For academic settings, make sure that the grading criteria include your priorities for the assignment.

Example of the Strategy at Work   During a summer discussion course I realized that formal lectures for every class would prove difficult for students and faculty alike. I composed a list of presentation topics equal to the number of students in the class and assigned two **Student-led Seminars** to each session. All topics began with the phrase "Nursing care of the client with_____." One presentation was given halfway through the class and one at the end. A brief discussion followed each presentation.

I told my students to adhere strictly to the time limit and to focus on nursing priorities and the implications of the condition. I instructed them not to discuss pathophysiology, elaborate laboratory tests or diagnostics, or in-depth management strategies. Instead, I asked them to briefly discuss the disease, nursing assessments, and any care included in the disease management.

Creativity, organization, ability to engage the class, and emphasis on priorities all counted toward the grade. I also asked for a reference list in American Psychological Association (APA) format that included at least three resources, one of which was a nursing research article mentioned in the presentation.

Table 4–2 shows the grading system I use for this assignment in a discussion group.

Students came up with many creative teaching strategies to enhance their classmates' enjoyment of the seminars. One student brought in an older adult relative. Simulating a client education session, the student discussed the client's nursing care and the assigned diagnosis. Another student prepared a presentation on sickle cell disease by baking cookies depicting sickled and nonsickled red blood cells. Another dressed in camouflage to discuss the role of chemotherapy in treating prostatic cancer. A student with computer skills created a newspaper with "articles" about the nursing priorities associated with the assigned condition. Videos, skits, food, costumes, and puzzles were only some of the strategies the class came up with.

Table 4–2. Student-led Seminar Topic		
Grading Criteria	**Points Available**	**Points Assigned**
Information is comprehensive and based on nursing priorities.	30	
Seminar is organized and adheres to time limits.	30	
Seminar includes creative strategies to engage class participants.	30	
Reference list is appropriate for APA format and nursing research article is appropriate.	10	
Total	100	

Ideas for Use

- As with **In-class Test Questions,** you can ask students in the audience to develop test questions about the seminar. These may be used in the review session or on actual tests to reinforce attentiveness during the seminars and encourage class attendance.
- If you draw test questions from the seminars, tell the class how many questions per seminar they can expect.
- Encourage students to develop a brief handout, like the **Legal Cheat Sheet,** for each of their classmates.
- Allow students a lot of latitude with their creativity to keep the assignment informative and fun.

Self-learning Mini-modules

General Description   **Self-learning Modules** are a well-documented strategy in nursing education.[16] To adapt them to an "on the run" strategy, I've created an abridged form of these modules.

Essentially, the instructor turns one small portion of the class into a **Self-learning Mini-module**. In the middle of a lecture, take a moment and pass out this mini-exercise to cover the next topic. The **Self-learning Mini-module** replaces the lecture for 5 to 10 minutes, and then the traditional class resumes. The content of the **Self-learning Mini-module** is not addressed verbally because the module is enough to convey the information. This strategy may be used in academic and continuing education settings.

Preparation and Equipment   The **Self-Learning Mini–module** consists of selected readings and questions, both of which you'll need to determine while planning your class. It's usually better to select a less complex topic for the module.

Example of the Strategy at Work   While covering nursing care of the hepatic, biliary, and pancreatic systems, I realized that class time was limited and that the hepatic system could take up most of it. I also noted that the biliary system discussion was largely related to the various terms used for biliary disease and management. I asked the students to bring their text to class and gave them an assignment similar to the one shown in Box 4–7.

Ideas for Use

- This strategy is ideal for an important subject that's a subset of a larger topic. The subject should be simple enough to teach by this method. **Self-Learning Mini-modules** emphasize the material without taking too much class time.
- Use this assignment as the **Admit Ticket** for the next class.

Box 4–7.
Nursing Care of the Client with a Biliary Disorder

In class, take 5 minutes and read (e.g., pp. 934–938) in your text. Then define the following terms:
1. Cholelithiasis
2. Cholecystitis
3. Choledochitis
4. Choledocholithiasis
5. Cholecystopathy

Now that you have defined the terms, indicate which of the following disorders in the left column match the assessment or management procedures in the right column.

1. Cholelithiasis	a. Cholecystogram
2. Cholecystitis	b. Choledochoplasty
3. Choledochitis	c. Cholecystectomy
4. Choledocholithiasis	d. Cholelithotripsy
5. Cholecystopathy	e. Choledocholithotomy

1 (e), 2 (c), 3 (b), 4 (a), 5 (d)

- Ask students to come up with their own mini-modules for class, study, and review sessions.
- Use case studies in your text to construct **Self-learning Mini-modules.**
- In academic classes, make sure the material covered in the **Self-Learning Mini-modules** is represented on tests.
- For continuing education settings, use this strategy to reinforce concepts and change gears. It can also provide a break for nurses not used to day-long classes or battling the after-lunch "sleepies."

Online Discussion Groups

General Description   The Internet provides several ways to communicate with students. The easiest way to conduct **Online Discussion Groups** is to use the agency server or platform for posting and receiving messages. Instructors post questions, and students participate in the discussion by posting their answers.

Online Discussion Groups stimulate critical thinking, personal problem-solving, and universal participation. Harden[17] demonstrated that these online sessions helped students better understand the material being discussed. In addition, they stimulated a positive exchange of ideas and a comfortable forum for sharing thoughts about nursing practice.

Within academic institutions, BlackBoard™ and WEB CT™ provide icons that lead participants into a discussion. Clinical agencies may already have, or can develop, a limited-access posting site for staff, new orientees, or unit personnel.

Preparation and Equipment   You'll need to access agency resources to make **Online Discussion Groups** work. Then you'll need to stimulate discussion or provide guidelines for the online groups. Some instructors participate actively; others "witness" or "observe" the discussion group. Either way, you can use the electronic platform to evaluate student participation and the quality of responses.

For academic instructors, evaluation and assignment guidelines should be part of the class syllabus. For agency instructors, **Online Discussion Groups** may be voluntary, to provide staff support and access to new policies and information, or may be a professional requirement.

Example of the Strategy at Work   In a large lecture class, stimulating meaningful discussion with all students may be a challenge. Even in smaller classes, total participation is difficult to attain. **Online Discussion Groups** provide an answer to this dilemma. I used this strategy in a winter class of accelerated (all second-degree and some second-career) nursing students. Weather constraints and other commitments made this group responsive to online discussion.

Each Monday and Thursday I posted a question to the discussion group. Because the winter session was condensed, the discussion sessions had to take place twice per week. Weekly or biweekly discussions would probably suffice for longer sessions.

I asked my students to respond at least twice to each discussion question, once by answering the question and once by responding to a classmate. After I set this parameter, it was interesting to watch the spirited discussions that followed my questions. Some questions stimulated a higher level of discussion than others, but I always felt rewarded at witnessing the level of thinking and passion in the students. Although I did not participate actively in the discussion, I often needed to alert the students to potential test material or provide a closure statement to summarize their observations.

Ideas for Use

- Internet etiquette, or "Netiquette," should always be respected and maintained. A fellow instructor and I meant well, but didn't know some of the rules associated with listservs in the early years. We asked students to sign on to a listserv, determine its purpose and view some of the key issues, and follow up with a reflective **Ah-hah Journal.** We heard from many listserv members that this use was not appropriate because listservs are meant for sharing specific information, not for education. We omitted this assignment, needless to say.

  It's important to tell your class that listservs are available to support nursing students. "Lists of lists," available on the Internet, can guide students in finding appropriate listservs.[18]

- Students also may be responsible for initiating **Online Discussion Groups,** establishing "thinking questions," and creating closure at the right time.

- Some Internet platforms provide chat rooms for real-time discussion. Chat rooms are a familiar resource for many students. However, students less used to computer chatting or instant messaging may need some orientation. Instructors can sign on to chat rooms at specified times to be available for questions or to set up an instructor-led discussion. The instructor can provide a virtual environment for post-conferences in clinical or discussion groups.

- Chat rooms and **Online Discussion Groups** are great tools for assessing the knowledge level of a class. Students can apply their problem-solving skills and explore class content.

- To make this an "On the Run" strategy, you can create mini-discussion groups for **E-mail Exercises** or **Ah-hah Journals.**

Learning Contracts

General Description   **Learning Contracts** enlist the students' contribution to their own course grade. This practice, especially common in nursing education outside the United States, is being used increasingly in this country. The instructor sets the course parameters and presents options for attaining specific grades, based on the completion of elective assignments. Returning adult and second-career students find **Learning Contracts** a valuable way to determine their own learning goals and to succeed in the course.[19]

Most **Learning Contracts** include the number of required assignments as well as the elective ones. Also included is the time frame for completion, instructions for achieving goals, and methods of course evaluation. A key element of the **Learning Contract** is student cooperation. Another is the instructor's explicit articulation of expectations—it's important to make sure everyone understands the contracts. Students agree to complete an anticipated number of assignments, but may change the contract as they wish during the semester.

Preparation and Equipment   To establish a **Learning Contract,** you need to delineate assignments clearly and explain the credit associated with each one. The class parameters, which allow students to determine their course grade, should be set out in the syllabus and policy statement. Establishing and maintaining **Learning Contracts** can be labor intensive and difficult. However, when students take responsibility for their own learning investment, the rewards are significant.[20]

Example of the Strategy at Work   A colleague of mine used a **Learning Contract** in a seminar course for senior nursing students.[21] Five assignments were required: a field trip, practice in standardized testing, weekly class activities, composing a resume and cover letter, and leading a small-group discussion. Completing all five assignments would ensure a grade of C+, four would bring a C, and three would result in a C–. Any student completing fewer than three assignments would fail the class. Each student signed a contract agreeing to these conditions.

In addition to these requirements, students were offered six optional assignments to raise their grades. These assignments included a field trip reaction paper (⅓ grade increase), a resume and cover letter resubmission (⅓ increase), an NCLEX® prep option (⅓ or ⅔ increase), political meeting attendance (⅔ increase), job fair attendance (⅓ increase), and a topic reaction paper (⅔ increase).

Ideas for Use

- **Learning Contracts** give students an effective way to control their grades.
- **Learning Contracts** reflect accomplishment and increase students' investment in their own success.
- **Learning Contracts** may be as elaborate or as simple as needed to meet the course objectives and the needs of the students.
- To make **Learning Contracts** an "on the run" strategy, you can let students negotiate and contract terms for specific assignments. For example, instructors may provide students with an array of several assignments to meet a course objective. Students may elect to write a paper, carry out a presentation, create patient education material, or another assignment. Key to this contract is to have students agree to a certain project and follow through, teaching another important lesson about commitment and obligation.
- Several resources document the feasibility of **Learning Contracts** for clinical groups in selected settings, including mental health and community health facilities.[22,23]

Condensed Portfolios

General Description   **Condensed Portfolios** can enhance a small class. In this strategy, students gather selected assignments and create a personal portfolio of their progress. These portfolios may be maintained on paper or electronically.

This strategy helps students assess their own performance and maintain personal records. They feel more responsible for preserving evidence of their performance and their attainment of course objectives.[24] Portfolios may include completed assignments and papers, clinical evaluation tools, anecdotal notes, reaction papers and journals, evidence of accomplishments, and formative and summative evaluations. They can be used for a single class or an entire curriculum.

Preparation and Equipment   Faculty need to establish clear evaluation policies for the use of portfolios within a course or curriculum. Individual instructors can add **Condensed Portfolio** expectations to their course syllabi. In agencies, orientation personnel can develop standards for nursing orientees to use in recording their professional growth. Agency portfolios might include records of attendance at educational programs, evidence that requirements have been met, certification documents, current resumes, and evaluations. As the literature confirms, the success of this strategy depends on clear guidelines related to expectations and portfolio contents.[25]

Example of the Strategy at Work   In an introductory nursing class, I asked students to create a personal portfolio of their progress through the course. As time went on, I adopted the name **Condensed Portfolios** to make it clear that these portfolios would contain only the information discussed in the course syllabus. By doing so, I eliminated a significant amount of extraneous information.

The course syllabus indicated the following contents of the *Context of Nursing Portfolio*:

- Responses to six **E-mail Exercises** with instructor comments. (Including these assignments gave students incentive to read my feedback.)
- The instructor-graded copy of the completed Nursing Database.
- The instructor-graded copy of the student's data-analysis project.
- The instructor-graded copy of the student's plan for client care.
- Evidence of a **Web Assignment** answering a class question.
- The instructor-graded copy of the American Psychological Association formatting exercise.
- Signed documentation of completion of Total Care Test-out, ensuring competency in basic care skill performance.
- The instructor-graded copy of the Nursing Economics Case Study.
- A final personal growth **Ah-hah Journal.**

This assignment was worth 10 percent of the course grade. Documentation of each assignment was worth one point except for the last assignment, which was worth two points. The extra point represented the amount of time students should have spent on the final **Ah-hah Journal,** which discussed their personal growth during the semester.

All the portfolio assignments had been required for the class; none were optional. I wanted the students to practice maintaining records, develop an organizational structure for the portfolio, and assume responsibility for completing it. These expectations fitted the objective of professionalism that underlies even a beginning-level nursing course.

Ideas for Use

- To establish **Condensed Portfolios** as an "on the run" strategy, you can develop assignments or policies aimed at creating an abbreviated portfolio.
- In nursing clinical groups, **Condensed Portfolios** can track individual progress through a rotation. Clinical evaluation tools, lists of

skills, and personal evaluation summaries can be included. Schools might establish policies allowing subsequent clinical faculty to assess student skills by reviewing these portfolios. The student's explicit consent would be needed for this use of the portfolio.

- You may want to develop assignments that build on one another and eventually become part of the **Condensed Portfolio.**
- Students can maintain a voluntary portfolio of their educational experience. They can show it to prospective employers or graduate schools, or use it for promotion within an agency.
- Agencies can use **Condensed Portfolios** in annual evaluations, as evidence for promotion or advancement in a clinical ladder, or as documentation for accreditation.

References

1. deBono, E: The Six Thinking Hats. Penguin Books, Markham, ON, 1985.
2. Gross, R; Peak Learning: How to Create Your Own Lifelong Program for Personal Enlightenment and Professional Success. Putnam, New York, 1999.
3. Sweeney, J, and Moeller, L: Decision training—The use of a decision curriculum with an in-basket simulation. Education 104:414–418, 1984.
4. Maslow, AH: The Farther Reaches of Human Nature. Viking, Oxford, England, 1971.
5. Bowles, DJ: Active learning strategies . . . not for the birds! International Journal of Nursing Education Scholarship 3(1). 2006 3:Article 22. Epub Sep 22.
6. Free, KW: What if? What else? What then? A critical thinking game. Nurse Educator 22(5):9–12, 1997.
7. Free, KW: What Next? Accessed from www.whatifgame.homestead.com. May 8, 2007.
8. Paul, D, and Elder, L: Critical Thinking Tools for Taking Charge of Your Professional and Personal Life. Prentice Hall, Philadelphia, 2002.
9. Krejci, JW: Imagery: Stimulating critical thinking by exploring mental models. Journal of the Organization of Nurse Executives 36(10):482–484, 1997.
10. DeYoung, S: Teaching Strategies for Nurse Educators. Prentice Hall, Upper Saddle River, NJ, 2003.
11. Rowling, JK: Harry Potter and the Sorcerer's Stone. Arthur A. Levine Books, London, UK, 1999.
12. Aronson, E, Blaney, C, Stephen, C, Sikes, J, and Snapp, M. The Jigsaw Classroom. Sage, Beverly Hills, CA, 1978.
13. Hunt, R: Readings in Community-based Nursing. Lippincott Williams & Wilkins, Philadelphia, 2000.
14. Mosteller, F: The "Muddiest Point in the Lecture" as a feedback device. The Journal of the Harvard-Danforth Center 3:10–21, 1989.

15. Oermann, M, and Gaberson, K: Evaluation and Testing in Nursing Education. Springer, New York, 2005.
16. Mast, ME, and Van Atta, MJ: Applying adult learning principles in instructional module design. Nurse Educator 11(1):35–39, 1986.
17. Harden, JK: Faculty and student experiences with web-based discussion groups in a large lecture setting. Nurse Educator 28(1):26–30, 2003.
18. Bridges, A: A "list" is not for groceries...A guide to electronic discussion groups in nursing. Journal of Nursing Administration 27(9):13–16, 1997.
19. Dix, G, and Hughes, SJ: Strategies to help students learn effectively. Nursing Standard 18(32):39–43, 2004.
20. Timmins, F: The usefulness of learning contracts in nursing education. Nursing Education in Practice 2:190–196, 2002.
21. Polek, C: Course Syllabus: NURS 460, Newark, DE: School of Nursing, University of Delaware, 2006.
22. Wai-Chi Chan, S, and Wai-Tong, C: Implementing contract learning in a clinical context. Journal of Advanced Nursing 31(2):298–305, 2000.
23. Watson, S: The use of reflection as an assessment of practice. Can you mark learning contracts? Nursing Education in Practice 2:150–159, 2002.
24. Ramey, SL, and Hay, ML: Using electronic portfolios to measure student achievement and assess curricular integrity. Nurse Educator 28(1):31–36, 2003.
25. McMullen, M: Students' perceptions on the use of portfolios in pre-registration nursing education: A questionnaire survey. International Journal of Nursing Studies 43:333–343, 2006.

Personal Journal Pages

Chapter 5

Strategies for Clinical Instruction and Orientation

> "I take one minute a few times a day to look at my goals and see what I want to learn .... I can teach myself what I want to learn more easily by taking one minute to catch myself doing something right. ... The more often we see the good in ourselves, the more we see the good in others ... the more often I have a good attitude, the more often I have a good day. We are at our best when

Challenges

- Clinical education, whether in an academic or an agency setting, is one of the most rewarding venues in which to pass on the craft of nursing. It also provides some of the greatest challenges in nursing education.

- Although the learning needs of new orientees and nursing students are important, the priority in a clinical agency is always safe and effective client care. Instructors struggle to balance client safety with the experiential needs of students. It can be especially difficult to foster learner independence in a clinical area.

- Instructors find it difficult to encourage critical thinking with a large number of students or orientees.

- Experiential learning creates a special kind of tension if some clients' conditions are more acute than others'. In such a setting, mistakes and inexperience cannot always be tolerated. This tension increases in environments with intense client needs, as in acute illness or injury. The nurse educator encounters demands in settings with poor staffing, in which nurses are constrained by frustration, or those who don't foster the growth of novice nurses. Clinical site shortages, lack of agency preceptors, and workforce issues exacerbate these problems.

- Instructors must encourage independence in their learners, whether staff or nursing students, while maintaining some sense of organization and control over the learning experience.

we teach ourselves what we need to learn." —S. Johnson and C. Johnson

- Evaluating student performance, whether for a grade or continued employment, is often difficult to balance with teaching. The question "When does teaching stop and evaluation begin?" can help instructors decide whether learners have met the objectives of the experience.
- The instructor may find it arduous to create a learning environment for multiple students with varying needs and skill levels.
- Pre- and post-conferences and learning debriefings usually take place before or after a hard day at work. It takes planning and effort to give these sessions value for the student.

Innovative methods can help you provide a safe and relevant education to novice nurses. In the clinical setting, you'll need strategies that foster learning in a tense environment; safe simulations outside of actual client care; and group exercises in which students learn vicariously through each other's experiences. Focus your strategies on critical thinking, priority setting, decision-making, and applying theory in the clinical setting. Clinical experience is one of the most valuable tools we have for teaching the nurses of tomorrow and those who already practice.

IDEAS

Scavenger Hunts

General Description   The primary objective of **Scavenger Hunts** is to help students get comfortable within their surroundings so they can work efficiently and effectively. One of the chief difficulties new employees encounter is not knowing where things are or how to access them quickly. This lack of knowledge may affect their ability to navigate both the physical environment and the virtual world of the computer. **Scavenger Hunts** provide a safe venue for finding, using, and understanding objects employed in daily nursing practice.

Preparation and Equipment   Although it takes a while to make up a **Scavenger Hunt,** the format may be used time and again to orient new students or employees to a clinical area. You can make up a list of five to six things to find or tasks to be completed in order to meet orientation objectives and develop a sense of comfort in the clinical area.

Example of the strategy at work   Box 5–1 shows the **Scavenger Hunt** I use for clinical orientation.

Ideas for Use

- **Scavenger Hunts** can be used in various ways to orient newcomers to a setting. Asking students to find things in the new environment develops their "search and explore" skills. You can ask them to find a straw, locate probe covers for the electronic thermometer, count the Band-aids® at the client's bedside, or hunt for other objects used in daily care.

- You can take **Scavenger Hunts** into the area of skills. Your students can learn to use objects they'll be responsible for in clinical practice. For example, you can ask students to take a tympanic temperature, take an electric blood pressure reading, find an empty crib or bed and raise and lower the side rails, or take their own oxygen saturation reading.

Box 5–1.
Clinical Scavenger Hunt

1. Find the tympanic thermometer on the unit. Take the temperature of a partner and record it here: _____ .

2. Find a drinking straw and record its location: _____ .

3. Access the electronic blood pressure cuff and take your instructor's blood pressure. Record it here: _____ .

4. Visit the dietary department and ask to see a low-sodium menu. Consider the lunch choices. Are soup or luncheon meats found on the menu? _____

5. Count the number of Band-aids found at the bedside of a client. Write the number here: _____.

6. Go to an unoccupied bed or crib. Attempt to lower the side rails. Note here whether it is harder or easier than you anticipated: _____

7. Ask the unit clerk to show you how to find clients' lab results. Record one client's most recent complete blood count here:

   _____

   _____

8. Use the computerized telephone directory to find the number for Spiritual Services. Record it here: _____

- You can help your students meet the people associated with the unit function. Ask the unit clerk which phone numbers are used most frequently and where to find the agency directory, how to transfer a call to another phone, or the procedure for printing lab results. Ask the unit pharmacist about the medications most often prescribed on a given unit. Talk with the dietary personnel about their customary times for tray delivery. Talk with a volunteer about his or her role on the unit.

- Some components of the unit may be especially conducive to **Scavenger Hunts.** You can plan searches through the code cart, the medication room, the supply closet, or the utility room. Other searches may be planned throughout the nurses' station.

- You can develop a great learning experience by involving a client's medical record in a **Scavenger Hunt**. Students can practice chart information retrieval by hunting for demographics, historical information, or current data before assuming responsibility for client care. Students should be reminded of the confidentiality of client information before this exercise.

- Enlist the support of your agency in developing **Scavenger Hunts.** Have students or orientees visit the pharmacy to retrieve an insert for a common medication administered on a unit, or stop by central supply to ascertain the cost of selected items. Send students to the medical library for information on a client's condition, to the lab for the latest clinical results, or to the dietary department to retrieve a menu for a specific medical diet. If you go this route, you'll need to spend a little time seeking the assistance of ancillary departments and making sure they won't feel burdened by sudden multiple visits.

- Develop a computer **Scavenger Hunt** based on all the principles I've discussed. Have students sign on to the actual medical record system or a demonstration unit to access specific client information. Ask them to retrieve lab results, admission dates, birth dates, number of scheduled and as-needed medications, or most recent medical orders. You'll be helping the students navigate a computer system and client database that are often unique to each clinical area and specialty. Again, client privacy should be reinforced before students access the client record system.

- Code, or crash, carts are frequently locked to ensure that they're stocked completely for emergency use. Create a virtual or video tour of the cart, showing each drawer and its contents as part of the presentation. Include a pre-test and post-test to measure competency in navigating the drawer.

- Compose a **Scavenger Hunt** that meets the specific needs of your clinical environment.
- It's essential to keep **Scavenger Hunts** both brief and fun. **Scavenger Hunts** that are too long or arduous will frustrate participants. You're simply trying to acquaint them with the environment enough so that the next time they need to find something, they'll venture into somewhat familiar surroundings.

Pass the Problem

General Description   I learned this strategy at a nursing education conference and have found it valuable for clinical groups, especially those new to care planning skills. Attributed to S. Kagan,[1] this strategy fosters thinking, team work, and planning.

First, I ask my students to take out a clean sheet of paper. At the top they write their client's age, sex, medical diagnosis, and a brief background description. Next, they write the primary nursing diagnosis to be used for their care plan. Then the fun starts—the paper is passed to each member of the clinical group. Each member is asked to contribute a client goal and a strategy for that nursing diagnosis.

Preparation and Equipment   This strategy needs very little preparation. You can develop a **Pass the Problem** form (Box 5–2) or just have students use blank paper.

Example of the Strategy at Work   I use the strategy as explained here during a clinical post-conference early in the rotation. Students are very creative with their ideas and the exercise often fosters a team spirit. Students and orientees learn vicariously about each other's clients because conversation always happens in response to this exercise.

Ideas for Use

- Keep the students to a strict time limit so they can all benefit from each other's contributions. I plan 4 minutes each for an eight-member clinical group, so we're are done in about 35 minutes. Usually students can make their comments in that amount of time.
- You can use any problem format you like to teach the **Pass the Problem** concept. Nursing Incoming and Outgoing Classifications (NIC/NOC), client problem lists, medical diagnoses, or patterns of function can also be adapted for use.
- Write **Pass the Problem** at the top of a sheet of paper, or use a form similar to mine, and give each student a copy. This gesture formalizes the strategy and gives it more credibility for some students.

Box 5–2.
Pass the Problem

Client: Age: Sex: Medical Diagnosis:
Background Information: _____

_____

Nursing Diagnosis:

Client Goal: _____
Nursing Intervention: _____

_____

Client Goal: _____
Nursing Intervention: _____

_____

Client Goal: _____
Nursing Intervention: _____

_____

Client Goal: _____
Nursing Intervention: _____

_____

Evaluation of client goals; effectiveness of interventions; revisions in care:

- You may want to review the format for client goals and nursing strategies before this exercise. It's important to make sure that students are clear on these concepts. Client goals are measurable, observable, realistic, and client-centered, with a target date. They should begin with the words "Client will . . ." Nursing strategies are individualized, realistic, understandable, specific, and nurse-oriented. They should begin with the words "Nurse will . . ."
- **Pass the Problem** is great for orientees using simulated clients and for teaching agency care plan formats. It promotes team

building; sharing of care plan skills; and assessment of individual knowledge about critical pathways, care plans, standards of care, and other planning formats.

- Students can get their papers back and spend a minute reviewing other members' contributions. Give them time to clarify information with each other.

- If time allows, encourage the students to relate interventions and goals to what they did or witnessed in client care for that shift. They can then evaluate goal attainment and effectiveness of interventions.

- Students and orientees can use **Pass the Problem** to plan care if they're assigned the same clients the next day. Other students may suggest new goals and interventions, enhancing the clinical experience and the client's level of care.

- Post-conferences and debriefings are a great time to complete this activity.

- You can use **Pass the Problem** in connection with the **One-minute Care Plan.**

Cooperative Strategies

General Description   An important skill for nursing students and new nurses to develop is teamwork. **Cooperative Strategies** build collaboration, not competition. They encourage the group to work together rather than in isolation. Foremost, they reinforce the knowledge that teamwork is a lifelong skill vital to professionalism in nursing.

Preparation and Equipment   The equipment needed depends on the emphasis of your **Cooperative Strategy.** By and large, this task requires a longstanding focus on teamwork and collegiality rather than specific supplies. The goal is to create a cooperative atmosphere that can translate to more effective and efficient client care.

Example of the Strategy at Work   On the first day of clinical work or orientation, assign pairs of students to take care of clients. Encourage students to assist each other, but not to overwhelm the client with their efforts. The students may take turns checking vital signs, cooperate during assessments so they don't duplicate efforts, and share in helping the client with activities of daily living.

Reinforce the concepts of delegation and cooperation in this first assignment. As time progresses, make assignments more challenging and independent, always asking students to solicit help as needed. To develop rapport, assign students to neighboring rooms in the early weeks of rotation or orientation. Encourage them to help each other, especially when client assignments are demanding.

Sometimes we praise students who function well independently. It's also crucial to reward teamwork in your evaluation of students and orientees. Recognize the importance of working together to accomplish goals.

Ideas for Use

- Cooperative games marketed for young children can set the stage for team building. There are no winners or losers in these games; the object is to work together for a common goal.
- Creative strategies described in other chapters of this book are great ways to begin team building in a clinical group, orientation cohort, or any other team in which work may reflect cooperative efforts. **Group Concept Mapping, In-Class Debates,** and **Group Thought** are effective ways to foster cooperation and teamwork.
- Show a film clip demonstrating team building, such as *Remember the Titans,* to demonstrate teamwork and collaborative nursing practice (see **Short Clips** and **Film Clips in Clinical**).
- If you encounter cliques, you may want to assign groups arbitrarily. You can use this tactic to pair more- and less-talented students and help them build on individual strengths. A student with a sound knowledge base but awkward interpersonal skills may complement a gregarious student who's less skilled in technical or analytical components.
- For nursing clinical groups, you can stimulate a teamwork spirit by such simple statements as, "We don't leave until everyone is done," and "We don't eat until everyone is ready." Students who finish an assignment early are encouraged to help the others so all can meet the common goal.
- Many agencies have client lifting and movement policies to prevent back and other injuries. Using **Cooperative Strategies** may help new nurses preserve their health as they develop good teamwork habits.
- Using pairs, trios, and groups within the clinical group can foster teamwork and collegiality.
- **Cooperative Strategies** encourage novice nurses to consider clients as partners, reflecting the current model of health care. **Grand Rounds, Clinical Quick Writes,** and **Day in the Life of a Client with . . .** may be used to reinforce this partnering message.

Here's a great **Cooperative Strategy** to read to a clinical group, especially one having interpersonal conflicts:

His name was Fleming and he was a poor Scottish farmer. One day, while trying to make a living for his family, he heard a cry for help coming from a nearby bog. He dropped his tools and ran to the bog.

There, mired to his waist in black muck, was a terrified boy screaming and struggling to free himself. Farmer Fleming saved the lad from what could have been a slow and terrifying death.

The next day a fancy carriage pulled up to the Scotsman's sparse home. An elegantly dressed nobleman stepped out and introduced himself as the father of the boy Farmer Fleming saved.

"I want to repay you," said the nobleman. "You saved my son's life."

"No, I cannot accept your payment for what I did," the Scottish farmer replied, waving off the offer. At that moment, the farmer's own son came to the door of the family hovel.

"Is that your son?" the nobleman asked.

"Yes," the farmer replied proudly.

"I'll make you a deal. Let me provide him with the level of education my own son will enjoy. If the lad is anything like his father, he'll no doubt grow to be a man we both will be proud of." And that he did.

Farmer Fleming's son attended the very best schools, and in time graduated from St. Mary's Hospital Medical School in London. He went on to become known throughout the world as the noted Sir Alexander Fleming, the discoverer of penicillin.

Years afterward, the same nobleman's son who was saved from the bog was stricken with pneumonia. What saved the man's life? Penicillin.

The name of the nobleman was Lord Randolph Churchill and his son was Sir Winston Churchill. What goes around, comes around.

Messages such as these stimulate thought. Discussion may be directed at developing positive relations among individuals in the group.

Clinical Quick Writes

General Description In this strategy, students are encouraged to develop and use writing skills to describe their experiences in caring for clients. **Clinical Quick Writes** may be done during conference or as an independent assignment. Several different versions of this strategy give students a safe opportunity for reflection.

Preparation and Equipment No specific preparation or equipment is needed. You should have a plan for the type of writing project to be assigned. Specific objectives and evaluation strategies should appear in the course guidelines.

Example of the Strategy at Work I have found this strategy especially valuable in post-conferences. After a long day of clinical work, students may find the post-conference tiring. Allowing time to write and vent some of the day's emotions provides closure and can make students more responsive to your feedback.

The most frequent **Clinical Quick Write** I use is "Write a Letter to Your Client." Students assemble in the conference room and get out a paper and pencil. They spend about 20 minutes composing a letter to one of the clients they took care of during the previous shift. Alternatively, they can write to a family member about their interaction with the client on that shift. This type of assignment is especially valuable in pediatric and maternity rotations, where family-centered care is very important. A colleague who uses this strategy in mental health care finds that it stimulates insight and builds empathy regarding psychosocial issues.

Ideas for Use

- You can assign **Clinical Quick Writes** as journal-keeping exercises.
- Ask students to spend a minute or longer writing down what happened during the shift. Obviously, this version is a true **Clinical Quick Write.** Students can use a narrative format to write about their day. Another approach is to write down as many words as they can to describe their experiences.
- You can ask students to write a single word or sentence that describes the clinical day. This word or sentence, shared with the group, generates discussion about the day, students' accomplishments, and goals for future clinical experiences. The conciseness of the exercise helps to focus thought and sharpen assessment and prioritization skills.
- The **Clinical Quick Write** strategy is effective for orientation groups, for team building, for a break in class or a change in atmosphere, and for dealing with controversial topics. For example, if a conflict occurs within the group, have all your students write down their thoughts. Let them choose whether or not to share them with the group.
- If a legal or ethical issue arises in the clinical area, students and novice nurses benefit from organizing their own thoughts. Reacting to the issue in writing may offer a chance for you and the group to discuss it. By having students write their personal reactions, you encourage participants to think about their progress and objectives for growth.
- **Quick Writes** help students explore personal issues about their profession. The strategy promotes a metacognitive approach, in which participants are asked to think about thinking.
- Provide the opportunity for a "free write" as part of the **Quick Write** exercise. Simply instruct the students to "write for 5 minutes." It's interesting to see what topics they choose and how they use this time as a chance for catharsis.

- You may use this strategy daily or weekly and keep the writings in the students' electronic or hard-copy folders. Students can review the file at the end of the rotation to appreciate their own growth and new breadth of experience. Assignments may be written on paper or submitted electronically.
- Ask the students to answer a written question or **Critical Thinking Exercise** in written format.
- If a troubling event occurred during the clinical shift, use post-conference as a chance for debriefing. Begin this session with private writing time. Conversation will follow from the students' reactions to their own and each others' writing.
- Always clarify whether **Clinical Quick Writes** will be private or shared. Writing may inspire personal reflections that students don't wish to make public.
- Use **Clinical Questioning** as a subject for **Clinical Quick Writes.**
- As I'll discuss later, keeping a journal is an effective way to focus thinking and investigate thoughts, emotions, and experiences.

One-Minute Care Plan

General Description   Many of us remember the elaborate care plans we produced in our nursing education. These long, detailed works drew on a plethora of sources and involved hours of work. Grounded in years of educational practice, this type of care plan provided an excellent learning experience. However, being specific to the care of one client and requiring a long preparation with extensive rationales, it lacks practicality in today's busy nursing practice.

The **One-Minute Care Plan** streamlines the time and pares down detail. This strategy gives students a useful and realistic means of organizing their thoughts, using the nursing process, and creating an accurate profile of a client.

Preparation and Equipment   You need to decide what client information is essential in clinical rotations. The setting, the objectives of the rotation or orientation phase, and your personal priorities can all influence your decision. You may assign the **One-Minute Care Plan** with explicit instructions or develop a form to be filled in like a worksheet. I've provided an example (Box 5–3), but you can make up your own or adapt this one for your needs.

Example of the Strategy at Work   I developed this form for my clinical groups after reading *The One Minute Teacher*[2] by S. Johnson and C. Johnson. This book is part of the "One Minute" series, and I recommend it highly. According to the authors, learning arises from the learner,

Box 5–3.
The One-Minute Care Plan

Client initials: Age: Medical Diagnosis: _____
_____

Brief Background Statement: _____
_____

Nursing Diagnosis:
_____
_____

Long-term Goal: _____
Short-term Goal: _____
Nursing Strategies:
   1. _____
   2. _____

Short-term Goal: _____
Nursing Strategies:
   1. _____
   2. _____

Nursing Diagnosis: _____
_____

Long-term Goal: _____
Short-term Goal: _____
Nursing Strategies:
   1. _____
   2. _____

Short-term Goal: _____
Nursing Strategies:
   1. _____
   2. _____

Evaluation of strategies and goal achievement:

and the teacher provides the framework for learners to teach themselves. The **One-Minute Care Plan** developed from that idea.

Ideas for Use

- Add medication sheets, lab data, and assessment information as needed to make sure the students have a good understanding of the client's condition.
- Use the following guidelines to ensure a comprehensive client profile:
  - Allergies
  - Diet (type and how tolerated)
  - Fluid requirements (based on weight and age or norms)
  - Reason for hospitalization
  - Other medical problems
  - Planned treatments (surgeries, therapies)
  - Current physiological status: Vital signs, pain status, oxygen saturation, review of systems
  - Lab and radiological findings
  - Current psychosocial status (fears, stressors, coping)
  - Family involvement (visiting, participation in care)
- Use this form during pre-conferences to prepare students for the clinical day. You may need to help students choose a nursing diagnosis; they sometimes have trouble anticipating nursing needs on the basis of a medical diagnosis or condition. Confer with them about care priorities, their role in the clinical experience, and their goals for the day for the client.
- Have students take notes on the form during report periods. I'm often surprised that when staff members give a report, students often either write nothing or write selectively. The **One-Minute Care Plan** may help them take down information that will affect care planning for their clients.
- Encourage the students to use the **One-Minute Care Plan** as a worksheet for ongoing assessments, developments in care, and news to be passed on in report. The strategy helps students decide "things to check," such as turning, medications, and scheduled treatments.
- This strategy also provides the framework for reporting to the staff. Students often just say to the nurses, "We're leaving," without realizing that certain information needs to be passed on.
- The **One-Minute Care Plan** allows students to reflect on the care they've provided and to think about potential revisions. After using the strategy to look back on the day, students can write in their

journals about objectives achieved, potential areas of concern, and personal goals for growth (see **Ah-hah Journals**).

- Establishing a system of organization is one of the biggest challenges for students and orientees. **One-Minute Care Plans** help them organize their day and their care. These plans can be adapted for individual and agency needs.
- Students caring for multiple clients may want to restrict their care plans to a brief client profile and one nursing diagnosis with goals and interventions.

Ah-hah Journal

General Description   The journal is a common method by which clinical instructors gauge student progress and get a "feel" for the student's thoughts and emotions. Less often, agency educators use it to assess the progress of new orientees.

The ease and perceived value of journal keeping varies among individuals. For some students, writing even five sentences is a painful experience. For others, page limits may be necessary to rein in their lengthy writing. The value of conventional journal keeping is questionable, especially if journals become chronological records of "things done" rather than "lessons learned." I still remember a five-page student journal that began, "At 6:45 a.m. I hung up my coat and prepared for my observation day in the ICU." Although this journal recounted every event of the day, it gave me no means of assessing critical thinking or any clue to the student's emotional side.

Hence the **Ah-hah Journal.** This strategy provides a glimpse of an event, giving some idea of the student's thoughts, emotions, and reflections on lessons learned during the clinical experience.

Preparation and Equipment   Put **Ah-hah Journal** guidelines in your class packet or syllabus. Assign a component of the class grade to this assignment, allowing for frequency, estimated page length, and the points assigned to the exercise.

For orientation groups, provide guidelines to validate the use of **Ah-hah Journals** as a legitimate way to document progress throughout the orientation period. Make sure you read all journals, comment about the student's observations, and demonstrate support of their reflective learning. Students provide more detail and share more readily when they think someone cares and is listening.

Example of the Strategy at Work   Box 5–4 shows the format I use for **Ah-hah Journals.**

Box 5–4.
The Ah-hah Journal

1. The Critical Incident (the episode or event)
    Note: The incident may be positive or negative
    A description of the experience including what happened, in
       sequence
    How and when the event started and ended
    A list and description of the people, things, or content
       involved in the event

2. Reaction and Analysis
    Your reactions, feelings, desires, and thoughts
    Nonverbal or other physical cues you noticed at the time
    Any associations while these reactions were occurring
    Examination of how you reacted to what happened and why
       these reactions occurred

3. Generalization
    Application of what was learned to future similar situations
    What you would change about the incident if it occurred again

Ideas for Use

- By describing events and thoughts, students are able to use **Ah-hah Journals** as learning exercises, which will help them generalize learned lessons to future events.
- By analyzing contributing factors, students learn to appreciate the complexity, and the often-competing priorities and perspectives associated with today's health-care environment.
- Make sure your students understand the format of the journal—it's not a record of the day or a validation of experience, but a reflection on lessons learned.
- Surprisingly, some students go through an entire clinical day and claim, "I had no **Ah-hahs** today." I always find this hard to believe. It's important for students to see **Ah-hahs** as both positive and negative, or even neutral, events. I tell students to think about the day and write about something they found surprising, or something they didn't know or hadn't thought of before the clinical experience.
   Michele Deck[3] describes "whack on the side of the head" experiences as those in which the individual is changed or

inspired by an event. Encourage students to find material for **Ah-hah Journals** in everyday life, and especially in their clinical work.

- For orientees, include **Ah-hah Journals** as part of weekly debriefings. Share common observations with the orientation group or allow orientees to disclose their own insights.
- **Ah-hah Journals** give you a great way to observe how students are doing in various sites or on different units. Observational experiences, such as the operating room, emergency department, and intensive care unit, are candidates for these journals.
- **Ah-hah Journals** let you "keep your finger on the pulse" of a clinical or orientation group. The process can uncover issues that require aggressive interventions, such as unit conflicts, staffing issues, or manager problems. This strategy can help you resolve conflicts sooner rather than later.

Creative Lab Skills

General Description   The nursing laboratory assists students to develop skills in dealing with heightened clinical acuity and more complex psychomotor skills. The number of nursing skills to be learned is always increasing. Nursing and staff development instructors must struggle to find effective teaching strategies that keep pace with the student's new level of learning.

Although a comprehensive discussion of teaching laboratory skills is beyond the focus of this book, several strategies can aid in teaching and reinforcing those skills. The emphasis is on learning the steps of a skill, understanding its scientific basis, and demonstrating it safely in the lab or the clinical area. Lab skills focus the sense of accomplishment for a novice nurse—competent completion of these skills gives students more satisfaction than other cognitive achievements do. For this reason, nursing instructors should be sensitive to the stress involved in learning motor skills. **Creative Lab Skills** help students learn them as thoroughly and expeditiously as possible.

Preparation and Equipment   Laboratory experience takes a fair amount of preparation. According to which strategy you use, you may need skills checklists, policy or procedure guidelines, and the equipment to practice the skills.

Example of the Strategy at Work   After growing numbers of students overwhelmed our old methods, our program searched for effective and cost-efficient ways to teach lab skills. Each course has certain skills assigned to it. Students attend the simulation resource center for practice and skill evaluation. The lab is staffed by a lab coordinator, who fosters the learning environment. Several aspects unique to our lab are noted in the Ideas for Use section.

Ideas for Use

- Audiovisual resources help in demonstrating lab skills. Use DVDs with both written content and movie clips. This approach appeals to diverse learning styles and allows you to repeat the demonstration.
- Each student purchases lab supplies in a duffel bag. The equipment company allows us to choose the supplies, which then belong to the student. The students can practice in the lab while you evaluate their progress. Having their own equipment also lets them try out their skills at home. This method is especially valuable for skills that take practice, like sterile gloving.
- A lab coordinator developed learning bins, which sorted the equipment needed for different skills. Students can use the contents as an adjunct to their personal equipment.
- Encourage the students to use peer teaching and learning as part of their lab skill training. Rather than demonstrating all the skills yourself, let the students actively coach each other using their skills textbook. Have them open the book at the mannequin's bedside and assist each other through the steps of a skill, providing feedback as needed. This peer teaching is valuable for both learner and coach. It ensures active integration of the skill, rather than the passive learning that follows a simple demonstration.
- Laboratory textbooks and checklists of skills are available from multiple publishers. You can either use these or make up your own checklists, though doing so can be very time-consuming.
- One faculty member suggested that students wear the school uniform when in the resource simulation lab. Uniforms foster a professional atmosphere in which the students "feel like nurses" and behave accordingly. Uniforms also help them regard the lab as an integral component of the clinical experience.
- Student teaching assistants have made a positive difference in our program. Having senior students assist junior students benefits both parties. More details about this program can be found in an article entitled "Benefits of Using Undergraduate Teaching Assistants Throughout a Baccalaureate Nursing Curriculum by Herrman and Waterhouse.[4]
- Actors posing as clients can be useful in teaching physical assessment skills to prelicensure students and advanced skills at the

graduate level. Schools may employ these actors or ask students to cover the cost as part of their course fees.

• For orientees and nurses new to a specialty, engage more senior clinicians to teach, assist with practice, and evaluate psychomotor skills. In clinical agencies with explicit procedure manuals, ensure that skills are taught and learned according to agency policy (see **Active Reading Conference**).

• The use of simulation mannequins has revolutionized the way nursing skills are taught in both schools and the clinical area. Simulators can be programmed to provide more than just a practice medium for a specific skill. They also can replicate a client's response in a given situation. Numerous resources exist for establishing and maintaining a simulation lab. Educational research has begun to develop an evidence basis for the use of simulators in nursing education across the practice field.

Equipment Conference

General Description   This strategy is just what it sounds like. **Equipment Conferences** acquaint students with equipment they'll use in the clinical area. Each agency has its own type of equipment, which may differ from what students used in previous lab work. This strategy reviews the basic workings of a piece of equipment and examines the nuances of a specific machine or set of supplies. Conferences take place away from the active clinical area. Thus they provide a safe opportunity to discuss the policies and procedures involved in operating and troubleshooting equipment.

Preparation and Equipment   Plan the time and place for the conference and bring the equipment with you. In some cases you'll need other supplies to put the equipment to work and allow students to practice.

Example of the Strategy at Work   Although students practiced clinical skills repeatedly in the lab, they consistently expressed misgivings about their skills. I chose to incorporate tracheostomy care and suctioning into their orientation day. We used several mannequins with simulated tracheostomies and portable suction to allow students to practice the skill in pairs.

The students practiced tracheostomy care according to the agency policy, which was slightly different than what they had learned in lab. They changed tracheostomy ties, did the suctioning procedure, and bagged the "client" to provide oxygenation between suctioning attempts. They rotated among the stations and practiced each skill. Students were encouraged to teach each other and provide feedback. An earlier tour of the unit had shown them how many clients were ventilated by tracheostomy. Seeing the wide clinical application of this skill helped them appreciate its relevance and immediacy.

Once I taught on an oncology unit, in which many clients had central venous access devices. One of our responsibilities was changing the central line dressings. We used the unit's format for teaching families: venous devices were accessed from staff development and inserted into placemats purchased at a local bargain store. The students brought central line dressing change kits to practice with. First, we all did the procedure together, discussing sterile technique, principles of asepsis, how to change a dressing on a moving client, and troubleshooting line complications. Then each student was able to change the dressing on an individual placemat.

In both examples, students were active during the conference period and reinforced a key skill for the clinical area. They could then be held accountable for that skill when the time came to provide it as a part of client care.

Ideas for Use

- Conduct **Equipment Conferences** early in the rotation to ensure competency before your students begin caring for clients. Start with less complex equipment, such as the pulse oximeter. Pass the sensor around the room to have students spot-check themselves. Move on to more complex skills throughout the rotation.
- If you can, obtain the equipment instruction manuals or agency policies to establish the procedures and show the students where they can obtain additional information about the skills.
- Identify the key skills the students will need on the unit: inserting Foley catheters, administering IV medications, using a feeding pump to administer tube feedings, using IV infusion pumps, caring for a client with a ventilator, changing complex dressings, and obtaining and interpreting ECG strips. These and many other skills can be reviewed in the clinical area if students' motivation is high and agency-specific equipment is available.
- Solicit feedback about what skills the students would like to review in conference time. As the rotation proceeds, poll them to find out what equipment or skills they find puzzling and build an **Equipment Conference** around those needs.
- Conferences may be held before, during, or after clinical or orientation days, or during other clinical meetings.
- **Equipment Conferences** may be instructor led or student led according to the needs of the group and the way students are evaluated. The **Equipment Conference** may be assigned to each student as part of the course grade.

- Enlist other professionals at the agency to help with **Equipment Conferences.** Respiratory therapists, dieticians, IV specialists, unit instructors, and staff development personnel can provide a high level of expertise concerning skills and agency-specific procedures.

Active Reading Conference

General Description   One surprise new nurses and nursing students face is the realization that there's more than one way to do certain things. Sometimes different procedures can accomplish the same skill with the same outcome. Another surprise for students and orientees is that clinical agencies have explicit procedures and standards of care, much like the skills texts and care plans used in nursing school.

The **Active Reading Conference** reveals the resources available in a clinical agency and reinforces the importance of those documents for safe practice. This strategy requires both students and faculty to be vigilant for frequently used skills or common nursing problems in the specific clinical area. The instructor assigns each student to seek out a procedure or the standard of care for that procedure. Students read this to the group during conference time. **Active Reading** calls for students to condense and summarize the information, making sure to emphasize key points, focus on nursing priorities, and allow for questions and comments.

Preparation and Equipment   Find the agency protocols and show them to the students early in agency orientation. Refer students to those documents frequently to ensure their use during clinical practice. Many agencies have converted their procedures and standards of care to an electronic format, available through the facility's network.

Example of the Strategy at Work   I was surprised to find that students often didn't know what resources were available. Then I realized that I, as their clinical instructor, was responsible for showing them these documents. That's how the **Active Reading Conference** was born.

A student needed to insert a nasogastric tube into a client and panicked. The student had learned the skill in the lab and been tested successfully—but now the time had come to really do it. We got out the agency manual, at the time bound in a notebook, read the procedure together, and completed the skill. The student, who marveled at the resource and how much it had helped with the task, wanted to share the experience in post-conference. The student copied the procedure and presented key points of the policy to fellow students while discussing the experience of inserting the nasogastric tube.

Ideas for Use

- Have students use a highlighter to emphasize key points of the standard of care or procedure before they present it to their peers.
- Tell students the point of the strategy—to emphasize key concepts and focus on nursing priorities. The word "reading" confuses some students, who think they're supposed to report on the document verbatim.
- Pass out company equipment handouts or other materials to help students learn about new equipment.
- Post **Active Reading Conference** information in the restrooms. One participant called this method "Elimination Illumination."
- This strategy can be incorporated into mandatory skills and orientation to ensure compliance with agency policies.
- The **Active Reading Conference** is especially valuable if the student assigned to read the case will be caring for a client needing this skill or care plan. Encourage the student to enhance the presentation with personal experiences. Students enjoy sharing insights—what it was like to do the procedure, the challenges encountered, and the sense of accomplishment following the task. The discussion can include client responses to the procedure and other nursing interventions, such as teaching, comforting, and client support.
- The **Active Reading Conference** may be effective in a service setting, where seasoned nurses forget the trepidation that skills can arouse in new nurses. Novices can share experiences and learn vicariously from each other.
- An important facet of this strategy is the legal and accrediting aspect of agency procedures and standards of care. Students also need to consider the ramifications of not knowing, not following, or deviating from agency protocols.
- Orientation groups can use this strategy to introduce procedures and standards of care to new employees. **Active Reading Conferences** or debriefings may be used to emphasize key skills and conditions the new nurse will encounter in the clinical area.
- Many organizations have their policies, procedures, and standards on their intranet, allowing students and orientees to download documents as needed.

Grand Rounds

General Description   **Grand Rounds** is a common strategy many of us remember from our days in school. However, some conditions have changed. Clients now expect to be informed about their care; at the same time, they expect that information to remain confidential. We've had to adapt our methods to meet the needs of students and orientees while respecting those of the client.

Grand Rounds requires each student to present cases either at the client's bedside or outside the room. Students are asked to provide a brief description of the client's issues and diagnoses, the course of treatment, and the nursing priorities and implications. An important component of this strategy is to seek the client's and family's permission before undertaking it.

Preparation and Equipment   No equipment is needed. You should preview the clients for whom students will present **Grand Rounds.** Higher acuity levels reflect an increase in the number of clients who may be too sick to qualify for this strategy. Students should understand how to speak about clients in their presence and what information to present. You can give them guidelines, such as a list of needed information: Client age, sex, and diagnosis; current course of treatment; nursing issues; and priorities at this time.

Example of the Strategy at Work   **Grand Rounds** is especially valuable when students have gotten comfortable caring for and interacting with clients. Toward the end of the rotation, they generally have the knowledge and poise to undertake the strategy. I let the students decide whether to conduct the **Grand Rounds** at the client's bedside or at the door.

I've also found it important to secure the permission of the nurse manager. Because of HIPAA and confidentiality restrictions, some leaders prefer that we use a conference room for these discussions. In such cases, I assign two or three **Grand Rounds** per clinical day. I ask all the students to introduce themselves to the clients we'll discuss that day, as well as to the clients' families. This tactic gives all the students a visual picture of the client to go along with the presentation. I also reinforce the need to be polite, caring, and respectful during all client interactions.

Ideas for Use

- Questions addressed in the **Clinical Questioning** strategy can become part of the student's presentation in **Grand Rounds.**
- Not only should we ask the client's and family's permission, but we should also ask their perceptions and priorities at this time: What is troubling you most? What do you expect to get out of this hospitalization? What do you need nursing to assist you with? These questions and others include clients as true partners in care.
- Some instructors find it valuable to include physical and other assessments as part of **Grand Rounds.** This method enlists clients' help in teaching the students or orientees. Again, it takes a special

client to agree, and the direction of **Grand Rounds** must change if the client becomes uncomfortable.

- Show the film clip from *Patch Adams* in which Patch so adeptly rehumanizes rounds by asking the client's name. Spend some time discussing that client's reactions to the other physicians and then to Patch as a way to model behaviors.

- **Grand Rounds** are meant to focus on client-specific information. This is not the time for elaborate discussions of pathophysiology or treatment options. For more in-depth discussions, see **One-minute Class** and **Student-led Seminars.**

- Students may share their **Ah-hahs,** their nursing priorities in the care of selected clients, and what they would do differently if they cared for the client again. This information must be shared judiciously if the rounds take place at the bedside.

- Use the **One-Minute Care Plan** to guide the structure of **Grand Rounds** if you would like to try a different format.

- **Grand Rounds** offers a great opportunity for students and orientees to present with knowledge and a sense of accomplishment. Talking about the client and answering questions gives students a chance to succeed and feel good about their progress. It's important for instructors to take a back seat at this time and allow the students to teach each other.

V-8 Conference

General Description   Students often focus solely on their assigned client or clients. In relation to other unit activities and to the experiences of other students, they sometimes seem to have blinders on. The **V-8 Conference** allows students to share experiences about their clients and to learn from each other.

Essentially, the **V-8 Conference** is a group-experienced **Ah-hah Journal.** Students share information that's newly learned, surprising, never thought about, or not previously known. The strategy gets its name from a familiar vegetable drink. The slogan "Wow, I could have had a V-8!" expresses an **Ah-hah.**

V-8 Conferences give students an opportunity to discuss their experiences and learn vicariously about clients or clinical issues. Keeping a 5-minute time frame, yet also allowing informal discussion, ensures that the entire group participates. The **V-8 Conference** may simply evolve in the direction of the conversation or may have a specific focus area selected by the group or the instructor. Students and orientees benefit greatly by hearing about the **Ah-hahs** of every member of the group.

Preparation and Equipment   Little preparation is required with this strategy. In fact, once the conversation is under way, you should provide very little input, allowing the students to lead the discussion. You may want to look over your available clinical days and select a focus to provide a direction for each **V-8 Conference.**

Example of the Strategy at Work   As a pediatric nursing instructor, I have two major goals in mind for clinical rotations. I hope that, in addition to learning safe, skilled, and organized clinical care, my students will embrace the concepts of *family-centered care* and *developmental care.* Because these are such high priorities of mine, I use two **V-8 Conferences,** one to address each issue. I present the topic at the beginning. Then the students discuss their personal observations and related client information in terms of their experiences. The assigned focus guides them in asking questions and relating facets of client care.

Ideas for Use

- You can assign a discussion group leader for the **V-8 Conference** or allow the leader to emerge naturally. Discussion leaders can be rotated to ensure equal participation and leadership experiences.
- A few possible topics are:
  - Family-centered care
  - Organizational skills needed to be a nurse
  - End-of-life care
  - Managing the critically ill client
  - Gearing care toward a client's developmental, not chronological, age
  - Clinical research protocols
  - Ethical issues in the clinical area
  - Delegation and working with unlicensed assistive personnel
  - Staffing and scheduling
- Use **V-8 Conferences** as part of the debriefing process during nursing orientation. Ask students to share their experiences and discuss common issues, frustrations, positive experiences, and areas for growth. Novice nurses may be relieved to learn that others feel the same way or confront similar stressors.
- Use **V-8 Conferences** as times to reinforce teamwork, collaboration, collegiality, mutual support, and learning. Foster problem-solving, decision-making, and critical thinking skills. Make sure the **V-8 Conference** doesn't become a complaint session, take on a competitive edge, or become a dreaded part of the clinical day.

- Students should see the **V-8 Conference** as their opportunity to learn and to talk. Intervene only if the conversation is inappropriate or contrary to the objectives of the clinical rotation.
- Conferences may be held before, during, or after clinical or orientation days, or during clinical meetings held at other times.
- Pre-conferences may take place before client care, when students are apprehensive, or after a hard shift, when they're exhausted. Either way, conferences need to be fun, creative, and informative. Encourage students to enjoy this time and see the value of sharing and learning together.
- Provide snacks or have a **V-8 Conference** during a meal time to foster a sharing atmosphere.

Documentation Case Study

General Description   The **Documentation Case Study** is one of my favorite clinical strategies. One of the greatest challenges for a nursing student or new employee is to master an agency's unique documentation procedures. Each facility has slightly different forms, expectations, and policies. In addition, different units, groups, or areas may differ subtly in what they mean by "note," "charting by exception," or "keeping up with your charting." Accrediting agencies have certain parameters for safe and legal documentation, but documentation guidelines may be interpreted differently within those constraints.

The **Documentation Case Study** was developed in response to these challenges. The case study is completed during clinical orientation and allows students to practice documentation skills before recording data in an actual medical record.

Preparation and Equipment   The **Documentation Case Study** is one strategy that takes a long time to develop. Once written, though, it can be used again and again. The strategy also makes it much easier to teach and learn agency documentation. First, you need to acquire the flow sheets, documentation policies, and other forms from the agency. Develop a case study and take the client through a care shift. As the shift proceeds, invent little detours that can present a documentation challenges. Develop the case with assessments, clinical information, interventions, and outcomes, all of which need to be documented.

You can be as creative as you like, Use this case and appropriate forms to construct an activity best conducted during the orientation phase of learning.

Example of the Strategy at Work   Here is the form I developed. Feel free to adapt it for your personal needs.

Documentation Case Study Exercise

Hello! You and a clinical group member have been assigned a complex case. In this exercise you'll work together to document the vital data you receive in your assessment. You may work together in any way you like.

You are caring for D.B., a client on the evening shift. He is a 3-year-old admitted for uncontrolled seizures and a history of asthma. On entering the room, you note that he is wearing his ID band and an allergy band indicating an allergy to adhesive tape. The side rails are up, a pulse oximeter is attached with the alarms on, and he is on seizure precautions. His family is at the bedside.

What precautions are indicated in a client at risk for seizure?

_____

_____

You note that his daily weight was not recorded on the day shift. During your assessment you weigh him; he weighs 31 lb. You need to record his weight in kilograms. His admission weight was 12.7 kg; his weight yesterday was 13.1 kg. At 1615 you proceed with the following assessment:

Vital signs: Temperature (axillary): 37.1, Heart rate: 105 bpm, Respirations: 20/min, Blood pressure: 87/56. He is on room air with an oxygen saturation of 89 percent.

Are these findings normal? What would you do?

_____

_____

At 1630 his work of breathing is increased with retractions. His breath sounds are coarse in the upper lobes bilaterally and decreased in the lower lobes, especially the left. He has a productive cough. You provide a prn aerosol breathing treatment of 2 mL metaproterenol with 1 mL cromolyn. You suction for a small amount of thin, cloudy drainage. You reassess at 1700 and find he had a positive response to the respiratory treatment.

What would you expect his work of breathing, breath sounds, and oxygen saturation to be after a positive response to the respiratory treatment?

_____

_____

You chart this respiratory response at 1700. Dinner has arrived. He is on a regular diet, eats well, and drinks 240 mL of juice and 180 mL of water.

How would you document his appetite?

At 1730 you move on with your assessment. You find that his color is pink, his skin is warm in all four extremities, he has no edema, and his pulses are strong in each limb. His capillary refill is less than 2 sec in the nail beds of his fingers and toes.

Is his capillary refill within normal limits?

He is able to follow your commands and assists you with your assessments. He has good muscle strength in his fingers, hips, and legs. His pupils are 4 mm, reacting bilaterally and briskly to lights.

Because of his episode of respiratory distress, he is placed on bed rest with bathroom privileges. He denies any pain. His belly is soft and flat and he has positive bowel sounds in all four quadrants.

At 1800, when you finish your assessment, he asks to use the bathroom. Measuring with a urine hat, you find he voids 75 mL of clear, yellow urine with a specific gravity of 1.030, negative for blood and ketones.

Is that specific gravity within normal limits?

What nursing interventions would you suggest?

At 1900 he has a formed small stool. You estimate it at about 50 mL. A HemaTest® is negative for blood. The stool is brown and formed, with a pH of 5. You give the child a complete bed bath.

The client does not have infusing IV fluids but does have an intravenous reservoir, to be flushed every 4 hours with 10 mL normal saline solution. This was done at 1900.

At 2000 he has a grand mal seizure lasting 45 seconds. You record it and the duration on the flow sheet. You document the description in the progress notes.

What behaviors would you expect to describe when documenting a grand mal seizure with full tonoclonic body movements?

After the seizure he vomits 10 mL of thick mucus. He is very sleepy postictally. He drinks 60 mL of flat cola at 2030 and voids 120 mL at that time, specific gravity 1.020. You prepare him for bed and assist him with his own oral hygiene. His vital signs at 2100 are:

Temperature (axillary): 36.9, Heart rate: 100 bpm, Respirations: 16/min, Blood pressure: 80/50. His assessment criteria for 2100 is the same as your afternoon assessment. Chart this assessment in the appropriate place.

His mother asks about seizure precautions and you provide teaching at 2130. Chart this in the progress notes.

As you prepare to leave the unit and report off to staff, you and your partner sign the flow sheet. Another busy shift!

Ideas for Use

- Use the **Documentation Case Study** early in orientation to teach important documentation skills.
- This exercise is a good way to reinforce the military 24-hour clock often used in clinical agencies.
- Have the students fill out the forms in pairs or trios, allowing for teamwork and team building.
- You may collect this form or allow students to keep it to use as a guide for future documentation.
- This exercise allows students to practice and make mistakes safely.
- The **Documentation Case Study** prevents a common error of new nurses—documenting just as the nurse before them did. Students and new nurses need to see the importance of valid documentation that reflects educated, thorough assessments and interventions.
- For observational experiences such as the operating room, postanesthesia care unit, intensive care units, and emergency department, obtain documentation forms and flow sheets to discuss with students. These will help to clarify the documentation processes in the different areas.

Clinical Questioning

General Description   Questioning students in the clinical area is a true art. It's not easy to catch up with eight to 12 nursing students or orientees, and difficult to assess their progress and preparation for clinical work. **Clinical Questioning** is a valuable tool you can use to determine a new nurse's readiness for increased challenge, safety in the clinical setting, strengths, and areas of future growth. This strategy is designed for the rapid assessment of individual progress. Alfaro-Lefevre[5] discussed the need for students to attend to three concepts in clinical thinking:

1. Thinking ahead (in preparation for the clinical experience)
2. Thinking in action (concurrently with client care)
3. Thinking back (reflecting on care delivered)

These concepts provide a framework for **Clinical Questioning.**

Preparation and Equipment Sage nursing instructors in both practice and academic settings can determine quickly when students or nurses are prepared, knowledgeable, and safe in the clinical area. They ask a few basic questions, honing in on clinical decision-making, assessment, and critical thinking.

As a clinical instructor, you need several of these questions "up your sleeve" in today's high-acuity health-care environments. Select and adapt the questions to the clinical unit or specialty and to your own style. Write them on an index card and carry it with you, tape to a clipboard, or memorize it. Have the questions available before or during client care. Use these questions readily with students to ensure their eligibility to provide client care. Tell your students that there may be more than one correct answer; this knowledge fosters critical thinking and creative problem-solving.

Example of the Strategy at Work Develop your own questions or adapt these:

What will you do today to make a difference in the life of this client?
What will you do to make your client better today?
What did you, or what will you, spend the most time doing today?
What one thing will you do differently the next time you take care of your client?
Why is *your client* on that medication?
How will you know the medication or treatment was successful?
What complications are you worried about with this client?
What signs and symptoms would indicate a deterioration of the client's condition?
How did you prepare to take care of your client?
What do you think concerns your client the most?
What information do you need to get from the client record as soon as you assume his or her care?
What three things that you heard in report will be priorities for you during your shift?

What three things will be most important to report to the staff when we leave?

What procedures and interventions did you witness that can be done in other ways? What aspect of the procedure would be different?

Ideas for Use

- Students generally find **Clinical Questioning** threatening and can feel judged. If you develop your questions in a nurturing, supportive manner, students will find it easier to express themselves articulately. Try to present **Clinical Questioning** as an opportunity for students to learn and demonstrate their level of knowledge.

- Ensure that students know your expectations for clinical preparation. Be clear about how much they should know regarding the disease process, medications, care plan, and client specifics. Emphasize that preparation for clinical experience is a professional expectation, not an option, and that it shows the nursing instructor that the student is ready to provide care.

- Make sure students know when to expect **Clinical Questioning** and how it will take place. A colleague of mine announces a set time before which students may solicit information from the client and staff, consult the medical record, and research questions. After that time, the student should be able to answer the instructor's **Clinical Questions.**

- Provide your **Clinical Questions** in the course materials or syllabus to make students aware of potential questions while they're preparing.

- Use **Clinical Questioning** to assess completion of orientation, achievement of objectives, and safety in the clinical area. Provide students with positive and negative, as well as formative and summative, information. Balancing teaching and evaluation can be one of the great challenges of clinical teaching. **Clinical Questioning** should be part of both processes.

- Use **Clinical Questioning** topics to shape student evaluations. Have students self-evaluate their performance using these questions as the basis for knowledge, preparation, and critical thinking. If you use objective evaluation tools to substantiate clinical performance, the focus stays on clinical course objectives and experiences during rotation.

- Make sure you don't single out any students during **Clinical Questioning.** The tendency is to assess weaker students repeatedly, which can make them feel "picked on." Offer the same amount of feedback to all your students, although its composition can differ drastically from one student to another.

Use the Book in Clinical

General Description   In clinical supervision, it's hard to keep up with what students are learning or have learned in didactic and previous clinical courses. Students sometimes deny experience or knowledge. They may feel overwhelmed, not wish to be held accountable, or truly forget some of the vast amount of information they've learned or heard in nursing school.

Use the Book in Clinical allows instructors, students, and orientees to consider what's learned in class and how it applies to the clinical area. Students bring their texts to the clinical area, look up needed information, and base conferences on their texts and other resources. This strategy also fosters inquiry skills, in which nurses actively research and investigate topics rather than simply learn by rote or authority.

Preparation and Equipment   Faculty who teach both clinical and didactic courses have a head start. Not only do they know what's being taught in class, they can help students apply that information to their clients. Part-time or exclusively clinical faculty often need to pursue such information themselves to know what's going on in the classroom. The same is true for agency staff development faculty embarking on creating a valuable orientation for a new employee.

All instructors should attend to the logic of the curriculum and think about how their courses fit into the total program objectives. Informal conversation with other faculty can clarify what clinical objectives, psychomotor skills, organizational abilities, and assessments students have mastered in previous courses. Course outlines and syllabi are useful. All faculty should have a copy of the textbook that corresponds to each clinical area. The text will show what students have read for class and how they're preparing for clinical rotations.

Example of the Strategy at Work   I **Use the Book in Clinical** continuously rather than as an isolated event. Clinical preparation is of paramount importance in safe client care. By knowing what's in their textbooks and remembering what has been discussed in their didactic classes, students can be held accountable and encouraged to apply their knowledge clinically. As classroom information grows more complex and students begin to care for high-acuity clients, it's imperative for them to make that connection.

Ideas for Use

- Before their clinical experience, students and orientees can present a client's medical diagnosis and nursing priorities using their textbook preparation. The presentation, which should be kept brief, may be done during pre-conference time.
- Staff development instructors may find it helpful to consult local nursing programs. They can provide valuable information about their curricula and show how students have learned from clinical experience at their agency.
- During conference, students can discuss what they learned in class about specific conditions, and can apply their knowledge to each other's clients. Your role is to make sure the information is valid and appropriate.
- Students have difficulty with the concepts of multiple diagnoses, comorbidities, and conflicting priorities brought on by severe health issues. They often expect a client to have only one diagnosis and become flustered with the complexity of the client's actual condition. **Use the Book in Clinical** helps students to unravel information and apply it to individual clients and their needs.
- Have both new and seasoned nurses peruse the textbooks on the unit. This tactic reminds them of lessons learned in nursing school and changes that may have occurred since that time. Reflection on their clinical learning can help them continue to learn and grow. Sharing textbook knowledge and experience can inspire discussion about practice issues, leading to **Research Moments** and **Clinical Area Questioning—Research at Work.**
- Use case studies, critical thinking exercises, and test questions in nursing texts to connect didactic learning with clinical practice.

Field Trips

General Description   We are all familiar with class field trips from our early school years. What we didn't always appreciate is that these trips were carefully planned around our learning needs. Similarly, **Field Trips** are a carefully planned facet of nursing clinical instruction. As is noted by Herrman, Saunders, and Selekman,[6] **Field Trips** are useful when additional experience is needed to complement what students customarily learn at clinical agencies.

Preparation and Equipment   **Field Trips** can take a considerable amount of planning or very little. Students may attend alone, in pairs, or in groups.

Example of the Strategy at Work   I experienced this strategy during my own nursing education. My instructor was way before her time. She contended that to provide holistic nursing care, students needed to be acquainted with the community and the neighborhood around the agency. She had us go to a local restaurant and arranged for us to be given a free portion of a local favorite food, visit the city hall and learn about the town, and window shop through local businesses to get a feel for the community. My students now use this "shoe leather" survey in wellness and community courses to get to know different communities and to learn about the needs of clients outside the agency.

Two ways I have used this strategy were in a pharmacology class. Students were asked to take two "field experiences." Here are the guidelines from their syllabus about these **Field Trips:**

Field Experience 1: Pharmacy Visit

For this assignment you can visit any pharmacy. Select an over-the-counter medication. Take a minute to read the label on the name-brand medication. Find the generic or store-brand medication and read that label carefully.

- Compare the ingredients of both medications.
- Compare the instructions given for both.
- Compare the packaging for both.
- Compare the prices for both.
- What important patient education issues are found on the medication labels?
- Is there a difference between the name brand and the generic or store brand?
- What is the reading level for both sets of instructions?
- Which medication would you purchase? Why?

Field Experience 2: Medicine Cabinet Assessment

Find a medicine cabinet that has at least six over-the-counter or prescription medications in it. Answer the following questions:

- List at least six medications in the cabinet.
- Are any of these medications expired?

- Are prescription medications in the originally labeled bottles?
- What specific precautions are noted for any of the medications?
- Imagine that a client is taking all six medications. What potential interactions should the nurse and the client be aware of?
- What safety issues might be associated with these medications?
- What client education issues can you identify?

Ideas for Use

- Arrange for students to visit and tour large metropolitan medical centers if current clinical sites are limited to community hospitals. Students learn a lot from **Field Trips** to emergency departments with helipads, large intensive care units, and specialty areas. Agencies with significant nursing workforce needs often use these tours for recruitment and marketing.
- Have students complete a community **Scavenger Hunt** as part of a **Field Trip.** As in my nursing school experience, arrange for them to visit local establishments and access local information to understand the community better.
- Pediatric nursing students can visit a toy store to learn about safe toys, developmental guidelines for toy choice, and how children play. If they compare prices, explicitness of directions, age recommendations, and safety aspects, they'll be able to provide anticipatory guidance for parents and caregivers.
- Pharmacology students can visit drugstores to peruse over-the-counter medications. Ask them to compare generic versus brand-name medications. Have them read the directions and determine the reading level of those directions. Ask them to consider the challenges experienced by people with visual impairment, for whom English is a second language, or with poor fine-motor skills. Their assessments can include medication administration instructions, childproof caps, and resources for people with low literacy skills or language disparities.
- Have students visit the local grocery store. Consider the needs of special populations, such as the elderly or those with disabilities, in navigating grocery stores with narrow aisles, carrying groceries inside the store and home, storing food, and preparing foods that come with complex instructions.
- As in the **Scavenger Hunt,** have students take a **Field Trip** within their clinical agency, such as to the medical library, the laboratory complex, or the research areas.

- One nursing instructor used a **Field Trip** to an art gallery to reinforce what the students knew about wellness and the role of nursing (Wikstrom[7]).
- Use shoe leather (walking) or windshield (driving) surveys for students to assess a community. Most community or wellness textbooks have a format for assessing a community's health. These can be adapted for the specific needs of the course and the clinical experience.
- Make sure **Field Trips** are objective driven and a necessary component of clinical education.
- Use **Injection Field Trips** to let your students practice giving immunizations. Contact a school health center, local affiliated health-care agencies, public health clinics, or local pharmacies for opportunities to give annual influenza injections. Students come away with a great feeling of accomplishment and skill mastery while providing a valuable community service.
- To bring home the challenges imposed by living in a wheelchair, one nursing instructor had students navigate the college campus in wheelchairs. Pairs of students, one in the chair and one assisting, experienced wheelchair accessibility or its lack, the reactions of others, and the environmental obstacles related to traffic, crowds, physical strength, and time constraints.
- Use **Ah-hah Journals** or **Online Discussion Groups** to evaluate the experience and students' levels of learning.

Learning From Each Other: Peer Teaching and Peer Team Leadership

General Description   In one of the quotations used in this book, Johnson and Johnson[2] state, "Everyone is both a student and a teacher." **Learning From Each Other** embraces that philosophy. In this strategy, instructors develop **Peer Teaching** and **Peer Team Leadership** activities in which students may assume the role of teacher. Students are assigned to these experiences on a rotational basis, allowing everyone to gain experience in leading and teaching others.

Preparation and Equipment   Assign students or orientees to both teaching and leadership roles during the clinical or orientation period. Students may be given some instruction on their role, methods of organizing data, and limitations on the role to ensure safe and efficient client care.

Example of the Strategy at Work

Peer Teaching

The **Peer Teaching** concept has been used a lot in nursing programs. Most programs require that a senior student be assigned to a junior clinical group for 1 to 4 days. During that time the **Peer Teacher** functions as an assistant nursing instructor, ensuring that tasks are completed, answering questions, and providing an extra pair of eyes and hands for the instructor. Before becoming **Peer Teachers,** senior students must complete the clinical rotation in which they'll be teaching and meet with the instructor to share expectations of the experience.

Students are often more comfortable asking questions of the **Peer Teacher.** In turn, **Peer Teachers** often feel a great sense of accomplishment when they can share what they know, realizing how much they've learned and grown during their time in nursing school. Nursing students often feel that there's always more to learn. As a result, they may lack a sense of accomplishment about their learning. This strategy gives them insight into how much they know and how far they've come.

Following the **Peer Teacher** strategy, the **Peer Teacher** and the students evaluate the experience and the individual students' levels of performance in both roles. The **Peer Teachers** may also self-evaluate and compare their teaching and leadership styles with those described in the literature.

Peer Team Leadership

The **Peer Team Leadership** concept is similar except that students from the same orientation or clinical group function as leaders for a specific period. They assist students with care, monitor task completion, ensure timely documentation, and seek out the assistance of the instructor as needed. This experience helps build organizational skills, models leadership behaviors, and builds rapport within the clinical or orientation group. Again, the evaluation of self and others is an important part of this strategy.

Ideas for Use

- This strategy is helpful for busy nursing instructors in high-acuity areas. It's important to remember that faculty alone are responsible for evaluating students. Also, agencies may have explicit policies about faculty supervision of students giving medications and completing skills.
- Clinical orientees may have a **Peer Teacher** or **Peer Team Leader** who rotates from among the nursing staff, increasing the rapport between staff and orientees and providing a mentor for clinical work.
- The **Peer Team Leader** may continue as a resource for new nurses who have just come off orientation. This tactic keeps a new nurse from feeling totally isolated in a newly independent role.

- Make sure that **Learning From Each Other** strategies breed team spirit and foster individual contribution. Students may become competitive in these roles, degrading group collaboration and individual feelings of success.
- Encourage students in the clinical area to **Learn From Each Other** by introducing each other to their clients and engaging in active discussions about client needs and nursing implications. Doing so encourages us to learn from our colleagues throughout our professional career.
- In classroom settings, encourage students to **Learn From Each Other** by setting up study groups, making up test questions for each other, and tutoring each other after they discover their strengths and areas for growth.
- Creative incentives—course credit, free parking, attendance at educational conferences, award certificates, credit for service learning or volunteer hours—may be given in return for tutoring services.
- Have students and orientees pair up—senior students or those who have cared for complex conditions should assist junior or new students. This method reinforces the teamwork inherent in nursing.
- Use **Pass the Problem, V-8 Conferences,** or the **One-Minute Class** to discuss common client issues, with the **Peer Teacher** or **Peer Team Leader** moderating the conversation.
- Solicit the input of the **Peer Teacher** or the **Peer Team Leader** to enhance student clinical evaluations.

Clinical Puzzle

General Description   I learned this strategy from a class participant. The exercise was developed as a playful activity for clinical groups, with each student responsible for a portion of the project.

First, the group chooses a client with a specific medical diagnosis or condition. Then, before the clinical day, each student is given a puzzle piece with a word or words such as *Nursing assessments, Lab data, History, Diagnostics, Medications/Effectiveness, Surgeries/Procedures, Discharge issues, Family issues, Developmental assessment,* and *Psychoemotional issues.* The number of students in the group will affect what's written on the puzzle piece.

Students use "down time" in clinical rotations to review the client's chart, consult other resources to investigate the condition, and talk with the client about the assigned aspect of care. Permission must be obtained before the students interact with the client. The instructor should take care not to overburden the client with too many eager students.

During post-conference that day or pre-conference the next day, students put the **Clinical Puzzle** together to create a comprehensive, holistic picture of the client and the medical condition.

Preparation and Equipment   Find a children's puzzle with as many pieces as there are students in the group. Writing the individual "assignment" on each puzzle piece is the only other task.

Example of the Strategy at Work   For the first clinical day in a rotation I generally assign students in pairs. This affords them more time than usual to research a client's condition and care. For the subject of the **Clinical Puzzle,** I select the most common diagnosis on the unit and a client with that condition. I don't assign any student to care for that client; all the students must start this assignment on an equal footing. I've used this strategy to help students understand type 1 diabetes mellitus and leukemia, but it's appropriate for many medical conditions.

Ideas for Use

- You can select the nursing or medical diagnosis most appropriate for the needs of the clinical unit.
- Students can research hypothetical or actual clients to complete the **Clinical Puzzle.**
- Monitor the students' work on this assignment to ensure that clinical work is being attended to. Also, the students' activities must not overwhelm the client or the client's nurse.
- Students need to see how each piece of information fits together to make up the client's clinical picture. A missing puzzle piece, just like a missing care component, skews the way we see the client and affects our care planning. To conclude this exercise, it's valuable to discuss how all the different pieces fit together.

One-Minute Class

General Description   Like the **One-Minute Care Plan,** the **One-Minute Class** gives students the opportunity to present a client to the group. The presentation must communicate integral information while filtering out anything extraneous. Although the talk may last longer than 1 minute, students are encouraged to condense information to provide a "snapshot" of the client in a brief period.

One of the greatest skills this exercise develops is the ability to focus. Essentially, students discriminate the "need to know" from the "nice to know." Only the highest priorities are discussed because there's no time for less important details—the student's day, the client's personality, or insignificant aspects of the client's treatment. This strategy differs from

Grand Rounds in asking students to focus on the nursing care and priorities identified in the **One-Minute Care Plan**.

Preparation and Equipment   Little preparation is required for this exercise. You can develop a format for the assignment or use the **One-Minute Care Plan** to guide the presentation.

Example of the Strategy at Work   Unlike **Grand Rounds,** which is most effective when the students are most knowledgeable, these strategies may be used early. The **One-Minute Class** and the **One-Minute Care Plan** complement each other and provide a means for students to organize their thoughts and their care.

During orientation I introduce the students to a client on the unit (after getting the client's and family's permission). I assess the client briefly and then leave the room (thanking the client and family again). I then pull the client's chart and show the students where to find the most information: the history and physical examination notes, the nursing database, and the progress notes. These sources give the students a glimpse into the medical record.

I pass out the **One-Minute Care Plan** form and we discuss the client's potential problems and issues. We discuss priorities and select two nursing diagnoses. I then verbally complete the **One-Minute Care Plan** form and demonstrate the **One-Minute Class.** Students are assigned to present their clients in the same way at subsequent conferences. Selecting a variety of clients will enrich the experience.

Ideas for Use

- Students can use the **One-Minute Care Plan** or **Pass the Problem** information as the basis for their **One-Minute Class.**
- For deeper pathophysiological perspective on the client's condition, see the **Student-led Seminar** For the client's personal experience, see **Grand Rounds.**
- The **One-Minute Class** may take place before the scheduled shift, when students are apprehensive about having to provide care, or after the clinical day, when they're exhausted after a hard shift. Either way, these conferences must be fun, creative, and informative. Encourage students to enjoy this time and see the value of sharing and learning together.
- Conferences may be held at any time and may even take place during clinical meetings.
- Orientees and novice nurses can use the **One-Minute Class** during their orientation period.
- You can use **Clinical Questioning** to form the structure for the **One-Minute Class.**

Film Clips in Clinical

General Description   As in the **Short Clips** strategy, film clips can reinforce concepts during clinical rotations. As we've seen, many films show content relevant to clinical issues. Showing a short clip and talking about it can generate discussion about issues outside a particular clinical area. If nothing else, **Film Clips in Clinical** provides a diversion from the usual conference format.

For this strategy, it's important to develop "thinking questions" based on clinical objectives, and to reinforce the nursing implications of events shown in the clip. Encourage your students to relate the **Film Clip** concepts to current clients, activities, and experiences. See Box 5–5 for potential thinking questions.

Preparation and Equipment   A laptop computer provides a portable, convenient way to show video footage. Clips saved to a CD or from a DVD may be shown to small clinical groups. Larger groups may need a VCR or DVD player (see **Short Clips** for details). **Film Clips in Clinical** should focus on clinical interactions, care of clients, legal and ethical issues, or other issues not always observable in the clinical area.

Herrman[8] has examined the use of films to enhance nursing education.

Example of the Strategy at Work   Table 5–1 shows some videos you can use to enhance clinical instruction.

Ideas for Use

- Make popcorn and show **Film Clips in Clinical** on the last day of rotations to end the experience on a pleasant note.
- Have students do a **Quick Write, Ah-hah Journal,** or **Online Discussion** to document their reactions to the clip and answer selected thinking questions.

Box 5–5.
Film Clips in Clinical: Thinking Questions

- How does this clip relate to our clinical experience?
- What is the role of the nurse in this clip?
- In this scene, what are the stated or implied nursing priorities for the clinical area?
- How will this clip affect your clinical care?
- How can you generalize lessons from this clip to future clinical experience?
- What are the nursing implications of this scene?

Table 5–1. Some Films to Use in Clinical Teaching	
Film Title	**Clinical Relevance**
As Good as it Gets (1990)	Obsessive disorder
	Myocardial infarction
	Interaction of sildenafil (Viagra) and nitroglycerine
Awakenings (1990)	Symptoms of extrapyramidal effects
	Frustrations of chronic illness
	Concepts of caring
	Inpatient psychiatric care
A Bag of Knees (2005)	Realities of nursing care
	Rewards of the nursing profession
	Survival skills for new nurses
A Beautiful Mind (2002)	Inpatient psychiatric care
	"Realness" of hallucinations and delusions
	Family impact of mental health issues
	Seizure activity
	Nursing process (separate clips to demonstrate each step)
Clean and Sober (1988)	Substance abuse
	Cross-addiction
	Denial of addiction
	Group counseling
Dead Poets' Society (1989)	Teen peer issues
	Teaching styles
	Group dynamics
	Emotional issues of adolescence
	Suicide and loss
Freaky Friday (2003)	Empathy—living the lives of others
	Mentoring
	Conflict resolution
How the Grinch Stole Christmas (2001)	Change theory
	Loneliness
	Caring

Continued

Table 5–1. Some Films to Use in Clinical Teaching—*cont'd*	
Film Title	**Clinical Relevance**
I Am Sam (2001)	Developmental disabilities
	Legal and ethical issues
	The judicial system
Iris (2001)	Progression of Alzheimer's disease
	Caregiver issues
	Disruption of family dynamics
	Nursing home care
John Q (2002)	Medical jargon
	Health-care financing
	Ethics in health care
	Use of technology in health care
Longtime Companion (1990)	AIDS
	Homosexual relationships
	Bereavement
Meet the Parents (2001)	Image of nursing
	Men in nursing
	Nurse–client interactions
My Flesh and Blood (2003)	Special-needs children
	Cystic fibrosis
	Severe burns
	Developmental disabilities
The Notebook (2005)	Dealing with aging
	Alzheimer's disease
	Loss and grief
	Frustration
October Sky (1999)	Teacher qualities
	Inspirational learning and goal setting
	Perseverance
Passion Fish (1992)	Quadriplegia following injury
	Stresses between client and caregiver

Table 5–1. Some Films to Use in Clinical Teaching—*cont'd*

Film Title	Clinical Relevance
Patch Adams (1999)	What not to do on rounds
	Humor in health care
	The mind–body connection
	Inpatient psychiatric care—group session
	Physical appearance of catatonia
Pearl Harbor (2001)	Depictions of pain and injury
	Nurses' role in World War II
	Response to death
Raging Bull (1980)	Head trauma
	Chronic traumatic encephalopathy
	Paranoia
	Physical symptoms of brain damage
Rain Man (1988)	Autism
	Developmental disabilities
	Family dynamics
Remember the Titans (2000)	Diversity
	Cultural struggles and awareness
	Teamwork
Save the Last Dance (2001)	Struggles of teen parenting
	Diversity
	Use of nursing theories to interpret issues
	Adolescence and issues with youth
The Sixth Sense (1999)	Children's perceptions of death
	Children's response to hospitalization
	Mental illness
	Parent interview in suspected child abuse
Steel Magnolias (1989)	Diabetes
	Chronic renal failure and dialysis
	Stress of pregnancy
	Family dynamics

Continued

Table 5–1. Some Films to Use in Clinical Teaching—*cont'd*	
Film Title	**Clinical Relevance**
Trainspotting (1996)	Heroin addiction
	Withdrawal symptoms
	Effects of addiction on family relationships
Wit (HBO Home Video, 2001)	Dealing with cancer
	Role of the nurse
	Interaction with the health-care community
Young Frankenstein (1974)	Communication techniques
	Injection techniques (improper)
	Teaching techniques
	Research and spirit of inquiry

- Show a clip and then have students play **Twosies** as a role-playing response to an interchange between actors. Ask students to rewrite the scene, making it more therapeutic or positive.
- Adhere to copyright and fair use laws while showing **Film Clips in Clinical.**

Make sure students see this strategy as a valuable clinical experience and not a frivolous exercise. Choose your clips and thinking questions carefully, keeping the course objectives in mind.

Let's Be Real in Clinical

General Description   Often the small size of clinical groups and the intense relationship with instructors lead to thought-provoking and emotionally charged discussions. **Let's Be Real in Clinical** helps an instructor mold these discussions into positive learning experiences.

Theoretical learning, preconceived notions about nursing, and workplace realities all come together in the clinical area. This part of a nursing student's education can be very stressful. Venting concerns and hearing the advice of a trusted mentor are as valuable as learning cognitive and psychomotor nursing skills. In this strategy, the instructor simply opens a conversation with the words **"Let's Be Real in Clinical."** The discussion that evolves may take many directions and contributes to the socialization aspect of nursing.

Preparation and Equipment   No preparation is needed. You merely set the stage and ground rules for open and honest communication.

Example of the Strategy at Work   I developed this strategy in response to a question I received from a student. During post-conference one day, I noticed that the entire group was exhausted. They had worked hard, learned a lot, and had little idle time to reflect on the day's events. In addition, they weren't looking forward to sitting for almost an hour in post-conference.

One student stated, "We were all so busy today. There were eight of us and six nurses and everyone was busy. How do the nurses do it when students aren't there to help out?" I suppressed a chuckle and the retort on the tip of my tongue: "Often staff feel they work harder when students are on the floor than when they're not."

Then I realized this was a great opportunity to discuss some of the realities of staff nursing. We discussed staffing, organizational skills, setting priorities, letting go of "nice to do but not necessary" tasks, and gaining nursing competence through experience. The students discussed these topics in light of the day's experiences, moving on to include their perceptions of reality from both class and clinical work. **Let's Be Real in Clinical** sets apart a time to voice concerns and discuss the realities of nursing from a personal and a professional perspective.

One question I like to ask involves the role of nursing in the health-care system. It's often said that nurses have a difficult time defining what we do. To glean students' perceptions I ask, "If nursing were to disappear tomorrow, what would be missing?" This question stimulates much discussion on the place of nursing in health care, the historical development of the nurse's role, and what role nurses will play in the future.

Ideas for Use

- Select questions to open the **Let's Be Real in Clinical** discussion, such as:
  - How do nursing staff manage multiple client needs?
  - How is the staffing different on off shifts, weekends, and holidays?
  - How do families handle the complex care of clients at home?
  - Will I be able to do this?
  - Is NCLEX® really that hard?
  - What are my job options in nursing?
  - How should I decide where to work after graduation?
  - How do people work and live with that disease?
  - How do I talk with clients about sex and sexuality?
  - What about nursing care is most important to me?

- What nursing specialty appeals the most to me?
- What issues affect the smooth management of a nursing unit?
- How do I care for clients who have value systems different from my own?
- What characteristics do I value most in a nursing leader?
- Do I want to pursue a higher level of education in nursing?
- Why do some nurses leave nursing?
- What are the pros and cons of 8-, 10-, and 12-hour shifts?
- What skills do I bring to nursing that guide me toward a certain clinical area or specialty?
- What qualities do I value in selecting a nursing mentor?
- Why do they say nurses eat their young?
- What are the staff's perceptions of nursing students in this agency?
- How has the nursing shortage affected the role of the nurse?
- How have the costs of health care affected the role of the nurse?
- How do policies and politics affect the role of the nurse?
- How are clients different now than 10 years ago?
- What legal and ethical challenges does nursing face in the coming years?
- How will advances in medical technology be reflected in nursing care?
- Do you prefer the "high-tech" or the "high-touch" components of nursing care—and are they mutually exclusive?
- These questions and a **Let's Be Real in Clinical** discussion give students the opportunity to vent fears, seek information, and share experiences. The strategy enhances team spirit and fosters greater cooperation in the clinical group.
- **Let's Be Real in Clinical** discussions may be adapted for **Online Discussion Groups, Ah-hah Journals,** or **Quick Writes.**
- This strategy is well received at the end of a clinical rotation or orientation period, when trust is high. **Let's Be Real in Clinical** provides a transition to the next clinical experience or to independent nursing.

References

1. Kagan, S: Cooperative Learning. Resources for Teachers, San Juan Capistrano, CA., 1992.
2. Johnson, S, and Johnson, C: The One Minute Teacher: How to Teach Others to Teach Themselves, William Morrow/Quill, New York, 1986.
3. Deck, ML: Instant Teaching Tools for Health Care Educators, Mosby, St. Louis, 1995.

4. Herrman, J, and Waterhouse, J: Benefits of using undergraduate teaching assistants throughout a baccalaureate nursing curriculum. 2007, in review.
5. Alfaro-Lefevre, R: Critical Thinking and Clinical Judgment: A Practical Approach, ed 4. Saunders, St. Louis, 2006.
6. Herrman, J, Saunders, A, and Selekman, J: Beyond hospital walls: Education pediatric nurses for the next millennium. Pediatric Nursing 24:96–99, 1998.
7. Wikstrom, BM: Nursing education at an art gallery. Journal of Nursing Scholarship 32(2):197–204, 2000.
8. Herrman, J: Using film clips to enhance nursing education. Nurse Educator 31(6):264–269, 2006.

Personal Journal Pages

Chapter 6

Strategies for Discussion Groups

"Shared perspectives, shared knowledge, and shared experiences are the key foundational building blocks of creativity."—Joseph S. C. Simplicio

Challenges

- Discussion groups present challenges similar to those encountered in both large and small classes. Discussion groups are usually smaller than regular classes, with only 10 to 20 participants.

- Smaller groups in academic environments may be graded for participation. The instructor must differentiate valuable contributions from those thrown in merely to gain credit. All participants must have an opportunity to add to the discussion. Sometimes the instructor has to address the problem of students who dominate the conversation.

- Smaller groups can challenge an instructor to maintain a learning pace and keep up interest in the topic. A smaller group may actually be more difficult to teach than a larger one. Such groups are often informal and may lack a concrete agenda.

- The influence of group dynamics may be especially pronounced in small discussion sessions—friendship ties and personal preferences rise to the surface and interfere with group cohesion and functioning. The instructor may have to provide more guidance than usual to ensure a positive learning experience for all members.

- Students who don't understand the material, or who are less gregarious, may find it even harder than usual to participate when the focus is on personal learning and growth.

- New nurses and orientation groups may be reluctant to participate, especially if they are worried about their new jobs, their personal growth needs, or how few people they know. Strategies to enhance comfort and group work are imperative with these smaller groups.

Group learning and innovative strategies can help to deal with these challenges. Discussion groups are a great way to clear up ambiguities, clarify difficult material, and address personal questions. Creative methods may assist in building a team focused on learning and succeeding in both personal and group goals.

IDEAS

In-class Debate

General Description   This strategy simply asks students to plan and carry out a debate discussing the pros and cons of an issue. The subject of the debate should be relevant to class objectives and may be selected by the students or assigned by the instructor. The instructor specifies the amount of detail in the exercise and how much class time it should take. In an academic setting, the elaborateness of the debate reflects the percentage of course credit given to the assignment.

Preparation and Equipment   The only preparation required for this assignment is the development of a list of debate topics.

Example of the Strategy at Work   I've used **In-class Debates** mainly in clinical post-conferences, although any small classroom setting is appropriate. One of our debate topics was a child in our care who was ventilator dependent, demonstrated little brain function, had no family support, and was sustained by gastrostomy tube feedings. The child had been born with very little brain structure, had a poor prognosis, and had been cared for by many of the nursing students. The nurses on the unit told the students that there had been much discussion at many levels about withdrawing ventilatory support and enteral feedings. The students expressed concern over the legal and ethical implications of this scenario.

For our post-conference we decided to have a debate rather than the student presentations already scheduled. Six students had not yet presented their seminars and agreed to take part in the debate. With three on each side, the students presented the case, debated the pros and cons of maintaining or withdrawing the medical regimen, and discussed the nursing implications of this type of issue. The experience was extremely valuable for everyone in the group. It felt especially poignant because of the students' intimate contact with the client and their personal investment in the case.

For discussion groups, I've needed to address assisted suicide as part of class content. **In-class Debate** contributions counted toward the group participation grade. We then used the statements in Box 6–1 to stimulate

Box 6–1.
A Right to Assisted Suicide

- Clients have the right to participate in all decisions related to their health care.
- Clients have the right to refuse extraordinary treatment.
- Comfort measures should always be provided.
- Clients have the right not to be interfered with in a rational act of suicide.
- Refusing life-sustaining measures is a form a suicide.
- Health professionals should always do their best to sustain a person's life.
- Health professionals have a responsibility to assist in a client's wish for suicide.

discussion and spontaneous debate. After a short class on legal and ethical decision-making, we switched gears to focus on each participant's thoughts about the statements.

As you can imagine, these statements generated a lot of thought and, as the questions became more complex, a significant amount of controversy.

Ideas for Use

- Extemporaneous speeches may be based on class topics. They may be as short as 3 to 4 minutes. Students pick a topic **Out of a Hat** and rapidly compose a debate position speech. Another class member is selected to take the opposing position. Finally, the class discusses both sides of the topic and class participants voice their personal opinions.
- This is a great method for enhancing class participation; usually quiet students may have a strong opinion about a "hot" topic.
- **In-class Debates** can occur spontaneously as controversial topics arise in class. Students can take their personal positions on an issue and provide their own arguments for or against it. **In-class Debates** are a great way for new or practicing nurses to begin clarifying their values related to practice issues.
- This exercise has a particularly challenging version: you can ask students to debate the opposite side of their personal beliefs. By taking a stand for the "other side," they must stretch their boundaries and carefully consider the pros and cons of the issue. In mounting their case this way, they're required to use true critical thinking.

- Students in discussion groups may be asked to debate each other and be peer graded on how convincing their presentations were. You may assign groups or allow the students to select their own.
- Some "real world" topics for debate may be:
  - Nationalized versus commodity-based or privatized health-care provision
  - The pros and cons of a practice seen in the clinical area
  - The nurse's role in administering a placebo medication
  - The role of a nurse who discovers that a fellow nurse is abusing substances
  - The use of restraints in a clinical agency
  - Methods of delegation and associated legal issues
  - The pros and cons and the realities associated with cross-training (orienting to multiple specialties within an agency) and pulling (routing staff to unassigned units to meet staffing needs)
  - The nurse's role when informed consent is lacking
  - The role of a nurse who believes a client has been coerced
  - What is considered professional in nursing uniforms
  - Any other controversial topic with an arguable pro and con
- For students who don't wish to participate in an **In-class Debate** or where a debate is not feasible, assign a **Clinical Quick Write** or a **Write to Learn** exercise. Other possibilities are an **E-mail Exercise** or a debate during an **Online Discussion.**
- Clinical and orientation groups may enjoy using the debate format to discuss their previous experiences and the protocols or philosophies of their new agency.
- In a practice setting, use the **In-class Debate** format to guide the development of standards, to address organizational policy changes, or to discuss the adoption of a controversial practice. This format allows all sides to be heard and ensures that the issue will be deliberated carefully. In the **Six Hats** strategy, students use the debate template to take on varying roles in a discussion.

Teaching Trios

General Description   This strategy has students break up into trios. Many of the exercises discussed in this book, such as **Twosies, Think-Pair-Share, Clinical Quick Writes, Skits, Invented Dialogues, Nuts and Bolts, Active Reading Conferences,** and the **One-Minute Class** may be used with trios.

All three members of the trio may be active in this exercise. Alternatively, two participants may take a primary role and the third person act as witness or observer, evaluating the interaction or playing "fly on the wall." **Teaching Trios** are great for teaching life skills, such as conflict resolution, assertiveness, stress management, decision-making, and dealing with difficult people or situations. In both its forms, the strategy helps all three trio members understand what it's like to participate in all three roles.

Preparation and Equipment   This exercise takes a fair amount of planning to keep it in line with the class objectives. You'll need to make up a role for each member of the trio, and enough trios to represent a variety of client issues. You can write each role on an index card. Although it takes time to do this initially, you can use the cards again and again if you remember to collect them at the end of the exercise.

Example of the Strategy at Work   I use **Teaching Trios** to emphasize the role of the nurse as teacher. After the students split into trios, each one gets an index card with a role written on it. These roles are not shared with the other group members. Each student tries to play the role dictated by the card.

After 1 minute each student passes the card to the next student: whoever had card One now has card Two, and so on, for 1 minute. Then they pass again. In those 3 minutes each student has been both a teacher and a learner with a specific learning challenge. For the final 2 minutes, the students discuss the difficulties they encountered during the exercise, the challenges of the varying tasks, and their responses as they played the different roles. Following are several examples of the trios I've used.

TRIO A

1. You are a nurse teaching a client to give himself insulin injections.
2. You are a 68-year-old client with diabetes, retinopathy, and poor vision.
3. You are the daughter of a client with diabetes. You have three children, a very demanding job, and multiple life stresses.

TRIO B

1. You are a nurse trying to go over a written set of discharge instructions with a client.
2. You are a client who is unable to read and too ashamed to admit it.
3. You are an observer who is aware that the client is unable to read and won't admit it.

TRIO C

1. You are a nurse practitioner teaching safe sexual practices to a young, sexually active male client.
2. You are a 16-year-old who is having a sports physical and admits to having unprotected sex.
3. You are the mother of a 16-year-old boy who, as far as you know, is not sexually active.

TRIO D

1. You are a preoperative care nurse instructing a child who is having surgery in 1 week.
2. You are a 3-year-old child.
3. You are the mother of a 3-year-old and you are very nervous about your child's impending surgery.

TRIO E

1. You are a nurse teaching an Asian client that he must not take certain herbs because of a known interaction with the medicine prescribed by his physician.
2. You are a 55-year-old Asian man who strongly believes in the benefits of Eastern medicine.
3. You are the son of the client and believe that Eastern medicine is "hogwash" and that everyone should use Western medicine.

TRIO F

1. You are a school nurse teaching a 13-year-old and his mother about the use of his inhaler.
2. You are a 13-year-old bilingual boy embarrassed by needing to use an inhaler.
3. You are the mother of a teenager and speak no English.

TRIO G

1. You are a hospice nurse teaching a client and his son about comfort measures for the client, who is dying of cancer.
2. You are an 85-year-old man with very little will to live.
3. You are a 45-year-old man who is unwilling to admit that his father is terminally ill and wants all heroic measures taken to keep him alive.

TRIO H

1. You are teaching a woman the exercises she should do to facilitate recovery after a mastectomy.
2. You are a 42-year-old women who underwent a radical left mastectomy for breast cancer 4 days ago.
3. You are the husband of a woman who has had a mastectomy. You are appalled by her appearance and are worried that she will notice your reaction.

TRIO I

1. You are an outpatient oncology nurse teaching a client about the side effects of his chemotherapy treatment.
2. You are a man with cancer. You are devoutly religious and believe that "God will heal me, I don't need medicine."
3. You are a wife of a client with cancer and heartily believe in the medical advances that treat the disease.

TRIO J

1. You are a nurse in an HIV clinic teaching a client about blood-borne exposure and ways to keep sexual partners safe.
2. You are a homosexual client who has just found out he is HIV positive and doesn't want his partner to know.
3. You are the partner of a gay man and have no idea why you are at a clinic.

TRIO K

1. You are a staff nurse teaching a student how to complete a technical procedure. You believe in short cuts to get the job done.
2. You are a nursing student who has never done a certain procedure before.
3. You are a nurse watching a teaching session between a staff member and a student. You disagree with the methods used by the staff nurse.

TRIO L

1. You are a triage nurse in an Emergency Department teaching a client about injury prevention. The client has been to the ED six times in the last year with various minor injuries.
2. You are a 35-year-old woman whose husband beats her regularly. He always makes sure the injuries are minor and has threatened your children if you tell anyone.
3. You are a 40-year-old man with an 18-year history of alcoholism who believes that "what goes on in my house is my business."

Ideas for Use

- For large classes, make up about 10 packs of three cards each. Have the class discuss the various difficulties they encounter in trying to teach "clients" with differing challenges.
- Ask the students to discuss their challenges and potential nursing interventions related to learning impediments (e.g., language barrier, cultural beliefs, poor vision, developmental issues, illiteracy, lack of motivation).
- **Teaching Trios** are good practice for dealing with sensitive client issues. Examples of these are death and dying, sexuality, the nurse-student relationship, abusive situations, client advocacy, and conflicts involving spirituality.
- **Teaching Trios** may be used in a clinical group when students encounter a situation they don't know how to deal with or in which they feel uncomfortable.
- Students learn basic critiquing skills by playing the observer and commenting on other students' responses. Because the roles rotate, everyone gets this opportunity. Nurses and nursing students are notoriously "nice" and uncritical of each other. Providing guidelines for peer review is an important lesson for professional practice.
- Like many role-play exercises, **Teaching Trios** provides a "safe" environment for practicing skills and is well worth the preparation time.
- **Teaching Trios** permit role playing in a comfortable setting because the cards are passed quickly and each member takes a turn at each role.

Same Information

General Description Empathy and decision-making are two of the nursing skills we try to cultivate. These skills are based on the ability to embrace the context and complexity surrounding an issue. **Same Information** provides two different versions of a case study. Two groups are formed and each gets one study. Now comes the fun: a key feature of this strategy is that the students don't know there are two different versions of the case study.

Preparation and Equipment   Compose both versions of your story. It's easiest to write the shorter story and then think up the second part, which adds a little twist. This second part may be as short as a single paragraph. Make sure the story is aligned with the objectives of the class.

Example of the Strategy at Work   Split your group in half. Give the first case study to one group, and give the other group the same case study with the information you've added. Then ask the students to read the case and come to some conclusions about the circumstances.

The case below was used to teach a conflict resolution class for staff nurses. I'm sure you can imagine that the two versions stimulated some healthy discussion. As the discussion went on, the students understood that they were "dealing from two different decks of cards." **Same Information** demonstrates how unknown details and contextual factors may influence behavior, and how important it is to know the whole story before passing judgment.

Case One

You are a nurse working on a unit. You are making up the schedule for the winter holidays. The custom on the unit is to work every other holiday and to rotate Christmas and New Year's Day in alternate years.

A nurse comes to speak to you about Christmas. She has been working with you for 1½ years, worked on New Year's Day last year, and tells you she can't work on Christmas for personal reasons. She asks you to schedule her for this New Year's Day and not tell anyone.

Case Two

You are a nurse working on a unit. You are making up the schedule for the winter holidays. The custom on the unit is to work every other holiday and to rotate Christmas and New Year's in alternate years.

A nurse comes to speak to you about Christmas. She has been working with you for 1½ years, worked New Year's Day last year, and tells you she can't work on Christmas for personal reasons. She asks you to schedule her for this New Year's Day and not tell anyone.

After some discussion, you find out that she is a single parent and that her husband died 3 years ago around Christmastime. Her 9- and 11-year-old children have had a hard time adjusting to the holiday ever since. She is willing to work all the summer holidays. Although she has shared this information with you, she is a private person and asks you to keep it confidential.

You can imagine the colorful discussion about responsibility, taking turns at work, professionalism, empathy, and collegiality. When the information in the last paragraph emerged, the **Ah-hahs** drove home many points about context and knowing the "big picture."

In another class I was discussing congenital heart defects in children. I discussed the fact that rheumatic fever is often the sequela of untreated bacterial infections. We examined some reasons why an infection would go untreated: the infection is undetected, children do not receive antibiotics, and others. Several students raised the issue of a family's withholding antibiotics for a streptococcal infection, putting a child at risk for rheumatic heart disease. Following are the stories I composed for a subsequent class.

Case One

You are caring for a 6-year-old boy. He is being treated for rheumatic heart disease following a streptococcal infection. He has sustained significant valvular damage that may require corrective surgery. You note in the chart that the client was seen in a doctor's office and that antibiotics were prescribed 5 weeks before this admission. The parents deny filling the prescription and offer no explanation for their refusal to treat the infection.

Case Two

You are caring for a 6-year-old boy. He is being treated for rheumatic heart disease following a streptococcal infection. He has sustained significant valvular damage that may require corrective surgery. You note in the chart that the client was seen in a doctor's office and that antibiotics were prescribed 5 weeks before this admission. The parents deny filling the prescription and offer no explanation for their refusal to treat the infection.

When you enter the room the 6-year-old is surrounded by his family. You learn that the family has eight children and that two grandparents live with them, making a total of 12 people in a three-bedroom home. The father has recently been laid off from his job on the assembly line at an automotive plant. Although his health-care coverage continues, they no longer have a prescription plan. The parents elected not to fill the prescription because the family is trying to make ends meet. The grandmother has many folk remedies that have served the family well for generations, so the parents have decided to treat the infection "our own way."

These scenarios highlighted the need to ask questions, rather than make assumptions, about situations. We then discussed the need for health-care personnel to explain why it's important to follow a care plan. In this case, the nurse should use explicit rationales and explain the potential complications of not treating the condition. The family should also receive help in finding appropriate community resources. The strengths of this family must be emphasized while the child receives the best treatment available. This important lesson is difficult to describe without the use of such a story.

Ideas for Use

- Use **Same Information** when students find it hard to understand another point of view or appreciate extenuating circumstances.
- Have students compose their own **Same Information** scenarios with specific objectives in mind.
- Make up a case any time to teach the value of perspective and the need to know the whole story before passing judgment.
- In leadership classes, this strategy is valuable for teaching decision-making and helping participants "see the forest despite the trees." If different parties don't have the **Same Information,** or if management bases decisions on unknown factors, new leaders often encounter frustration. This exercise illustrates the need to understand the "big picture" and respect decision-making while adhering to personal principles.
- **Same Information** is an effective approach to such topics as cultural and spiritual diversity, different values, attentive listening, and respect for individual beliefs.

Think-Pair-Share

General Description   **Think-Pair-Share** is most valuable when used with other strategies. Its name describes it well: first the students **Think** about an issue, then they **Pair** up, and finally they **Share** their thoughts.

In this strategy, first described by Lyman,[1] student pairs may share their observations with the larger group or not. Contributing factors are class time, class size, and the intricacy of the material. The key part of this strategy is the opportunity and time to contemplate the exercise and then share it with a partner. Students can pair with a neighbor or pick another partner, or you can assign partners. **Think-Pair-Share** partners may be assigned for a single exercise or for the duration of the class.

Preparation and Equipment   You'll need to decide the partnership terms and create the **Think-Pair-Share** exercises. It's important that the students "buy in" to the value of pairing and sharing, and that they not use the time for personal conversations or extraneous talking.

Example of the Strategy at Work   In this strategy I often ask students to look at a single statement, think about it, and offer comment. These statements resemble those used in **Why Are You in Nursing and Other Mysteries?, Critical Thinking Exercises, Past Experiences with . . ., What's the Big Deal?, What's the Point?, Clinical Decision-making Exercises,** and **E-mail Exercises.** Box 6–2 shows examples of some **Think-Pair-Share** statements.

I've also used this strategy as a basis for class exercises. Pairing off the class gives me a small enough group to work with and ensures active participation from everyone. Students often can get into pairs and begin

---

Box 6–2.
Think-Pair-Share

Name the Legal Infraction
- A nurse decides to put a client in restraints so he doesn't have to worry about him at night.
- A nurse is supposed to turn a client every 2 hours, but does not.
- A nurse gives a client an extra dose of sedative to "keep her quiet all night."
- A nurse removes narcotics from the unit narcotic cabinet and takes them during her work shift.
- A nurse documents that he has assessed the client's IV, but he has not.
- A nurse tells her neighbors about a client who had a therapeutic abortion on her unit.
- A client decides to withdraw from a research study, but health-care personnel will not allow it.
- A person falsifies records to say that she is an RN, but she is not.
- A nursing student gives medication to the wrong client.

the activity faster than creating groups of larger numbers of participants, encouraging the time spent on task. **Think-Pair-Share** also reinforces the need to think individually and share perceptions. In this way, it differs from **Twosies,** in which students simply pair up and work on a task.

Here are two **Think-Pair-Shares** I use to teach conflict resolution and leadership styles. Effective in both large and small groups, they reinforce material rather than simply presenting it. The third exercise, a hypoglycemia case study, may be adapted for any diagnosis or client issue.

Conflict Resolution Exercise

You are an Assistant Nurse Manager of a medical-surgical unit. Two nurses you work with on the unit do not get along. They ignore each other when working together, gossip about each other behind their backs, and do not communicate important client information. One day Nurse A accuses Nurse B of neglecting an important task required for client care. Then Nurse B accuses Nurse A of "spying on" her and "having it in for" her. Nurse A says she is concerned about care; Nurse B feels that Nurse A is being picky. How can you help resolve this episode?

Each pair is assigned a conflict resolution approach and given the following instructions: Come up with a solution to this situation based on the assigned method. What will you do to resolve this conflict? How effective do you believe you will be? What method do you think would be the most effective?

Collaboration: Both sides of the conflict work together toward a solution that does not deny the rights of either. The resolution is fully satisfactory to both sides and is a win-win situation.

Compromise: Both people sacrifice something so they can meet in the middle and agree on a solution. This situation is often described as lose-lose because neither side achieves an optimal solution.

Accommodation: This is a win-lose situation in which one person gives in to the other for the sake of a quick resolution.

Competition: In this approach both people assert their own needs and deny the other person's desires completely. This is another win-lose situation, in which resolution is accomplished through "survival of the fittest."

Avoidance: The conflict is denied and "swept under the rug." Neither person behaves assertively and the problem is left unresolved. Alternatively, each student pair can respond in all five styles and then conjecture which style would work best in that situation.

Leadership Exercise

You are an Assistant Nurse Manager delegating work during your assigned shift. You notice that one staff member doesn't seem to be completing tasks, does not interact with clients, and only briefly reports off to staff. Other staff members have noticed, but no one has attempted to resolve the situation.

Each pair is given a leadership style. Come up with one quotation, comment, or technique that represents your assigned leadership style:

Autocratic
Democratic
Charismatic
Laissez-faire
Situational
Transformational

Students then come together to share each leadership style, response, and rationale. First each pair, and then the larger groups, try to reach a consensus about which style would be most effective. Students don't always agree on a style. The difference in their opinions demonstrates the plurality of leadership styles.

Hypoglycemia Case Study

You are caring for an 8-year-old with diabetes. After he returns from physical therapy he complains of feeling shaky and weak. It is 10 a.m., and you know the dietary department has brought his morning snack. His 7:30 a.m. blood sugar was 458 mg/dL and his urine was negative for ketones at that time. He is now looking diaphoretic and seems tired and listless.

1. What is the first thing you should do?
    Check his blood sugar.
2. What issues might you need to explore?
    How much insulin was used to correct the 7:30 a.m. hyperglycemia?
    Did he receive insulin glargine (a peakless insulin) last night?
    Did he eat breakfast?
    How did he sleep last night?
    Did he work harder than usual at PT?

3. Should you recheck his urine?
   No, he is showing signs of hypoglycemia, not hyperglycemia.
4. Should he eat his snack?
   If his blood sugar is low, correct with 15 gm of carbohydrates and wait 15 minutes. If his level is still low, he needs another glucose correction.
   If his level is normal, he should have a protein and fat snack. Giving him his snack will also depend on its contents and his blood sugar level.
5. What, if anything, could have been done to prevent this episode?
   His doses of both a.m. and p.m. insulin should have been lower and he should have eaten more breakfast.
6. What will you do the next day?
   Give him a lower dose of a.m. insulin; reschedule PT so it doesn't coincide with the a.m. insulin peak.

Ideas for Use

- **Think-Pair-Share** is also a great icebreaker, encouraging students to talk and get to know each other more personally than the average classroom allows. Use the strategy when you sense this need in your classroom.
- **Think-Pair-Share** gives less gregarious students a private context for sharing their thoughts and insights about an exercise.
- Use **Critical Thinking Exercises, Clinical Decision-making Exercises,** or **E-mail Exercises** to provide the structure for **Think-Pair-Share.**
- Ask **Think-Pair-Share** pairs to compose a **Clinical Quick Write** assignment and turn it in for grading. You can also assign a peer evaluation, in which pairs trade off assignments.
- **Think-Pair-Share** is a great way to address legal and ethical dilemmas or areas of controversy. This strategy encourages students to think deeply about issues and to share their perceptions in a safe duo.

Admit Ticket

General Description   In this exercise, the assignment is to accomplish a certain task and provide physical evidence that the task has been completed. That evidence is the student's **Admit Ticket** into the classroom (Herrman[2]). The tasks and the **Admit Tickets** may take many forms.

Admission to the class depends on following instructions, completing the task, and remembering to bring the evidence.

Preparation and Equipment   You'll need to set aside a small amount of class time for this strategy. You must compose questions or solicit comments, making sure the assignment is clear. In case students show up for class without **Admit Tickets,** policies should be clearly delineated and enforced equally. The syllabus must be clear about both the assignments and the repercussions of not bringing the **Admit Ticket** to class.

For continuing education classes, you can use incentives to reward students who bring their **Admit Tickets.** This method precludes embarrassment and negative feelings for attendees who come without their Admit Ticket. It's important to remember that this strategy isn't meant to punish, but to reward going the extra mile in the learning environment.

Example of the Strategy at Work   I used **Admit Tickets** in a Friday afternoon class. My colleagues and I were having a hard time getting students to attend because they frequently worked, traveled, or had other activities on Friday. We used the strategy for students who attended class and stayed for the entire session, providing extra credit for each **Admit Ticket** collected. Although the amount of extra credit per assignment was very small, the accumulated points could affect the grade substantially.

Admit Ticket tasks included composing test questions, answering questions based on lecture content, developing a response to a "thinking question," and other tasks designed by the course faculty. In continuing education, we routinely require students to bring certain materials to class, especially in critical care, pharmacology, or resuscitation classes. Assigning these materials as **Admit Tickets** reinforces the importance of bringing them to class.

Ideas for Use

- Sometimes we feel that **Admit Tickets** work against us. Some nursing educators are so happy to have students attend class that we don't want to turn anyone away. We worry that students who are unprepared may just decide not to come. One instructor adapted this strategy from an **Admit Ticket** to an Exit Ticket. The students needed to answer a question or perform some other task before they could leave the class. Especially in continuing education, we want to reinforce class attendance and lifelong learning rather than dissuade them.
- Combine this strategy with **In-class Test Questions**. Have students make up test questions about that day's class and hand them in as an Exit Ticket or an **Admit Ticket** for the next class.

- **Admit Tickets** encourage attendance even when they aren't due. Students don't want to miss a class in which an **Admit Ticket** might be assigned for the next class.
- **Admit Ticket** may work better in smaller classes. Too many people can create a crowd at the door or make it unwieldy to collect tickets.
- Use **Admit Ticket** in combination with **Muddiest Part.** Ask students to identify the content areas they find the most confusing or complex and to write them on the **Admit Ticket** for the next class. Reviewing the **Admit Tickets** lets you assess the class and provide further instruction about difficult concepts.
- For continuing education programs, ask registrants to bring an **Admit Ticket** related to their objectives for the class (see **Why Are You in Nursing? and Other Mysteries**). Provide incentives. such as lunch passes or prizes. for those who follow through and bring the **Admit Tickets.**
- Certain **Admit Tickets** are required in some mandatory education classes, such as annual classes and resuscitation renewals. They include certification cards, completed pre-tests, and competency checklists. These demonstrations of personal responsibility reinforce the privilege of attending class and the professionalism associated with the learner's role.
- Combine this strategy with **Current Events.** As an **Admit Ticket,** have students bring in news clippings or downloaded copies of articles concerning health and health care.
- This strategy continues the socialization process by emphasizing personal responsibility. It also promotes active involvement in class and preparation for each session.

Write to Learn

General Description   This strategy is based on the premise that writing enhances learning. **Write to Learn** means just that—using writing assignments to help students learn and retain material. Those tasks can be as brief or elaborate as time and class objectives warrant. Instructors may assign the **Write to Learn** topic or allow students to write freely.

Preparation and Equipment   For academic settings, you'll determine the written assignment and your method of evaluating it. The syllabus should specify whether the writing exercise is to be graded or is simply a classroom teaching strategy. You may also decide to incorporate the **Write to Learn** assignment in the class participation grade; assignments handed in during class also provide an attendance record. For continuing education, **Write to Learn** is a valuable way to keep the class active and involved. Even if you don't evaluate the assignments, you can use them to assess understanding and attentiveness. Prizes can provide incentive to participate in **Write to Learn** activities.

Example of the Strategy at Work   **Write to Learn** is effective when several topics are discussed in a single session and time is at a premium. When teaching a class about eye disorders, I found that the students were puzzled by the differences between retinal detachment, glaucoma, and cataracts. They were especially confused by the differences between closed-angle and open-angle glaucoma. The **Write to Learn** I assigned was a 1-minute paper defining each condition or differentiating open- and closed-angle glaucoma. (A 1-minute paper is a quick writing assignment with a specific focus. The students actually had 3 minutes to complete the exercise.) Another few minutes were spent discussing their answers. I did not collect or grade the assignments, but assured the class that those concepts would appear on the examination.

I assigned another **Write to Learn** as part of a lecture on the nursing care of clients with neuromuscular diseases. Students typically have a tough time differentiating myasthenia gravis, Guillain-Barré syndrome, amyotrophic lateral sclerosis, multiple sclerosis, muscular dystrophy, and Parkinson's disease. These complex diseases, all with involved neurological, muscular, and orthopedic sequelae, are confusing and difficult to remember. Key knowledge for nursing students, though, is that the nursing priorities for these conditions are very similar.

After a fair amount of class time spent on the different diseases, etiologies, assessments, and diagnostic procedures, I assigned a 2-minute **Write to Learn** on the common nursing care priorities and interventions. As in **What's the Point?** or **What's the Big Deal?,** students wrote about issues in nursing such illnesses. These included airway, comfort, elimination, dealing with immobility, avoiding injury (e.g., aspiration, skin breakdown, falls), and emotional issues. I encouraged students to bullet or list their ideas and come up with as many issues as possible in the time allowed. We then discussed the commonalities and differences among the nursing priorities. The students benefited from the subsequent discussion, which explored the depression, frustration, loneliness, and anger that can accompany these conditions.

The assignments were handed in and included in the class participation grade. They also gave me an opportunity to assess the knowledge level of the class. Sometimes, because students get caught up in the need to memorize facts about pathophysiology, they need a reminder to focus on the nursing care common to many different conditions.

The last **Write to Learn** example comes from an elective course on adolescent health. We were discussing adolescent sexual activity and the pros and cons of abstinence-only versus comprehensive sex education for teens. The class started to evolve into an unplanned debate. Because I had a few very quiet students, I assigned everyone an individual **Write to Learn.** I asked them to spend 5 minutes writing down their thoughts on the topic and to substantiate them with personal experience or information. We then had a verbal **In-class Debate** with a high level of participation. The **Write to Learn** strategy allowed all the students to solidify their thoughts on the issue.

Ideas for Use

- See **Clinical Quick Writes** for the use of writing assignments in the clinical area. Writing a letter to your client, describing the clinical day or class in one sentence or word, or writing freely can also work in a classroom or discussion group.
- Writing in the classroom gives you an effective way to assess learning and comprehension. If you hit a **Muddiest Part,** you may want to take a few moments for a **Write to Learn.** It can help you determine whether you'll need to revisit the **Muddiest Part** in subsequent classes.
- **Write to Learn** exercises can be incorporated into **Learning Contracts.** Use the written assignments to gauge each student's performance against the standard work requirements.
- Discussion group participants can use **Write to Learn** to lay the groundwork for an **In-class Debate.** Students can write their thoughts about a controversial issue and then share in a debate format. The written precursor ensures that each student has thought about the issue and may have reached some conclusions.
- Continuing education students may not embrace the idea of **Writing to Learn** during a presentation. Keep written exercises short and fun. If you provide handouts, include a **Write to Learn** space so the exercise will look like a formal teaching strategy and not just a whim of the instructor.
- In general, include the **Write to Learn** question or topic in your handouts or audiovisuals to formalize the assignment and add credibility to your request.
- Use peer critique and grading on a set rubric. This tactic gives the students experience and eliminates the need for you to evaluate all the assignments.
- Have students **Think-Pair-Share** about each other's compositions.
- Ask students to summarize the main point of the class discussion in one sentence. For an easy **Write to Learn,** have each student complete the sentence "Today's class was about . . ."

- Provide a data set about a client or condition. Ask students to analyze it and come up with client issues and nursing interventions. Use this with **Pass the Problem** to encourage the class to share insights.
- For graded assignments, use a $0-1-2$ scale. 0 = not acceptable; 1 = acceptable but incomplete; 2 = acceptable and comprehensive.
- Here is a good exercise for beginning nursing students:
  - You are caring for a client in the clinical area. He refuses a bath for the third day in a row.
  - What rationale could the client have for his refusal?
  - What would you do?
  - What are the consequences of your actions?

Group Concept Mapping

General Description   Concept mapping is a well-documented strategy in nursing education. Beitz[3] gives a comprehensive review of concept mapping and its use in the learning process. The author specifically addresses concept maps and learning theory, concept map construction, the advantages and disadvantages of the method, and its application to nursing practice.

Concept maps are two-dimensional diagrams of a process, illness, concept, or construct. **Group Concept Mapping** is a slightly different version of this strategy: students in a discussion or clinical group work together to map an assigned or selected topic. The relationships between boxes or circles are established with connecting arrows (Fig. 6–1). These relationships illustrate the complexity and the interrelation of conditions the students will encounter in practice.

Preparation and Equipment   Little preparation is necessary for this strategy. You'll need to think of a study topic that relates to class objectives. For materials, you'll need large writing surfaces, large paper, and markers or crayons. This strategy can take some time, so students need to be clear about the time limit. Assigning the topic in advance gives them an idea of the main concepts to be mapped. If the assignment is being graded for an academic class, the details should be set out in the syllabus.

Example of the Strategy at Work   I used **Group Concept Maps** as a post-conference for a clinical group. The pediatric nursing faculty had agreed that students should assess each client's hydration status carefully and calculate maintenance fluid requirements according to their clients' weight. Students were puzzled about the priority given fluid status, which isn't an area of emphasis in adult nursing.

Fig. 6–1. Group concept map. Solid arrows show the interaction of risk factors. Dotted arrows show the nurse's conclusion based on assessment of these factors. BUN = blood urea nitrogen; I & O = intake and output; LOC = level of consciousness; NG = nasogastric; GT = gastrostomy.

We discussed the developmental and physiological characteristics that predispose pediatric clients, especially infants, to dehydration. I asked the students to research fluid status in children and be ready to do a project in the next post-conference. The **Group Concept Map** they developed is shown in Figure 6–1. In this map, fluid input and output and physiological function all influence the client's dehydration potential. Clearly, vigilant assessments can prevent future episodes of dehydration.

Ideas for Use

- **Group Concept Mapping** requires a significant level of cooperation within the group. It's a good way to develop or to retain team-building qualities.
- Develop concept maps for complex conditions seen in clinical settings, such as burns, congestive heart failure, chronic obstructive pulmonary disease, and diabetes.

- Concept maps can include physical signs and symptoms, precipitating factors, nursing diagnoses, discharge planning, risk factors, stages of illness, lab and diagnostic studies, medical and surgical treatments, and medications. The lines between components are important because they represent the establishment of relationships, a form of critical thinking.
- **Group Concept Mapping** provides a valuable review of conditions discussed in class but not encountered in the clinical area.
- Any medical or nursing diagnosis may be developed into a **Group Concept Mapping** exercise.
- Include a **Group Concept Mapping** assignment in your final evaluations of learning. Students will have to meet on their own time to complete the task and hand it in for grading.
- As in all group work, students must share responsibilities, delegate appropriately, and ensure total group participation. These lessons in themselves are a valuable component of **Group Concept Mapping.**
- In continuing education classes, use this strategy to teach complex algorithms and unfamiliar diseases or specialties.
- Everyone's idea of a concept map is different. With **Group Concept Mapping,** negotiation is a key element.
- Software is now available to create concept maps or mind maps. Standard word processing packages can also be used to develop them. Students generally hand in creative and attractive concept maps that reflect thought and hard work.
- See **Research Concept Maps** for details of using concept maps in research classes.
- The literature is replete with the use of individual concept mapping in nursing education.

War Stories and Clinical Anecdotes

General Description   We all have stories from our past. We tell them to relate experiences or illustrate important lessons we've learned. We also remember stories we were told to drive home a point or make an impression. Humans learn well by stories, especially auditory learners, who develop an internal "tape" of information they've heard.

War Stories and Clinical Anecdotes is based on these ideas. The strategy has become a common mode of teaching in the health-care field. The work of nurses and other health professionals, filled with human drama, real-life application, intrigue, and mystery, provides a fertile field in which to root our stories. People outside of health care are often fascinated by the life-and-death nature of our work, our view of people's intimate sides, and the miracles we perform regularly.

New students and nurses are just as enthralled by our stories. Because of the interest we stimulate and the memories we create, **War Stories and Clinical Anecdotes** is a stalwart of many nurse educators' portfolios. This strategy comes with some caveats, however. It's important to make sure your stories enhance retention and don't detract from learning or from other strategies. The key lessons should be clearly evident; this is not a time for hidden messages or covert lessons.

Preparation and Equipment   **War Stories and Clinical Anecdotes** may seem spontaneous and unplanned to students. In reality, personal stories should be well planned and should coincide with class content. Stories that stray from course objectives may mislead students and throw you off focus. They also take up precious time, limiting your ability to keep the class on schedule.

When you prepare your lecture on content, consider which **War Stories and Clinical Anecdotes** relate directly to the class. Which ones do you think of when you revisit the information? Make a few notes about the story in the margins of your lecture guide. Add two to three key words you'd like to use in retelling it.

It may also help to decide how much time you can devote to the story. One to two minutes will let you make a concise point without dwelling too long on a single incident. I've learned the importance of preplanning to make sure I include only the most relevant information and maintain the focus of the class. Marginal notes give me prompts for the components of the story I want to relay to the class.

Example of the Strategy at Work   Nursing instructors use **War Stories and Clinical Anecdotes** across the learning spectrum. Many of us remember stories from our education that have stuck with us for years. I've found that relaying stories from my childhood, education, early nursing practice, parenting experiences, and current life can trigger memories for students.

One story I've found useful comes from my early practice as a nurse. I was caring for a child who had sustained significant trauma in a motor vehicle accident. The child had been cleared of internal injuries and was stable. On the night shift, we were assessing his vital signs with neurological checks every 2 hours. The child rested comfortably between my visits with his mother at the bedside. He was voiding in his diaper and his assessments remained unchanged throughout the night—except for his heart rate, which increased throughout the shift.

I began checking his heart rate every hour. Worried that I was missing signs of pain, I carefully checked behavioral and physiological signs to assess his comfort level. I noted early in the morning that his heart rate was markedly above baseline despite no other change in vital signs or assessments. In my gut I believed something was wrong. I called the resident and reported the finding. The physician examined the child. We tested his hemoglobin and hematocrit and found them remarkably low. Despite no physical signs, this child was bleeding. He was taken to surgery soon after, all because of a subtle sign and regular assessments.

I use that story to drive home the importance of the gut feeling and of vigilant assessments for postoperative, posttrauma, or ill clients. That story reinforces the need for high-quality nursing care far better than a simple statement. It also reflects the independence of nursing assessments, especially on the off shifts.

Ideas for Use

- Establish a repertoire of stories for content you teach often. Ensure that the stories meet course objectives and are kept brief.
- Use caution when sharing stories about previous students, especially if a story is derogatory. Students may begin to feel like potential fodder for your stories and may resent hearing about others' weaknesses or mistakes. Even "I heard of a student who" stories may be offensive. Stories should have a learning focus, not a judging one.
- Gauge the audience for their ability to tolerate graphic detail. Nurses are notorious for gory, detailed work stories, even at the dinner table. Use your discretion to make sure your **War Stories and Clinical Anecdotes** don't horrify the students.
- Carefully weave the story into class content and objectives so students see the connection. It should be clearly evident and memorable.
- Make sure students comprehend that the story is only an example or prototype of the study topic. Novice students may generalize facts about your story to everyone with the same condition. They may have a difficult time transferring knowledge to the wide and varying array of human illness and trauma.
- Ask students, new nurses, and experienced nurses to share their **War Stories and Clinical Anecdotes.** As the class moderator, keep the stories on track. Make sure the sharing doesn't become a gripe session or a "Can you top this?" conversation.
- Use PowerPoint slides to provide visual prompts for the stories.
- Have students do a **Clinical Quick Write, Write to Learn,** or **Ah-hah Journal** in which they reflect on and derive personal lessons from your story.

Nuts and Bolts

General Description   **Nuts and Bolts** parallels the typical case study approach, with an added emphasis on fun and creativity. The difference between this strategy and a case study is what's missing: participants provide words to complete a story, focusing on the **Nuts and Bolts** of a situation. The format, shown in Box 6–3, recalls a familiar childhood travel game.

Preparation and Equipment   No preparation is needed for this exercise, although you may wish to show the format as a slide. You can interject **Nuts and Bolts** into any class to generate discussion about a condition and the related nursing priorities.

Example of the Strategy at Work   I've used this strategy in a class to differentiate the issues associated with left- and right-sided congestive heart failure. Students often have a difficult time understanding the similarities and differences between these conditions. See Boxes 6–4 and 6–5 for the two **Nuts and Bolts** stories I use to clarify these issues.

As students accrue knowledge and get the gist of the game, the underlined areas of each case may be left blank. Students can fill in the blanks by asking such questions as:

- What signs and symptoms would a client with this illness demonstrate?
- What are the initial nursing priorities?
- What is the medical treatment?
- How would you evaluate the effectiveness of the nursing or medical treatment?

The same exercise is used to differentiate hyperglycemia and hypoglycemia in Boxes 6–6 and 6–7. This distinction is a common subject of NCLEX® questions. Test participants analyze symptoms to determine high or low blood sugar levels and then decide the appropriate nursing interventions.

Box 6–3.
Nuts and Bolts Format

Once upon a time there was a _____ who had _____ and was _____ . The nurse assessed the client, determined that ____ had _____ , and began to _____ . As a result of the nurse's actions the client _____ .

Box 6–4.
Nuts and Bolts Exercise

Left Congestive Heart Failure

Once upon a time there was a *63-year-old man* who had *a history of chronic left ventricular congestive heart failure* and was *admitted to the unit with shortness of breath.* The nurse assessed the client, determined that he had *significant dyspnea, orthopnea, and an O_2 saturation of 83%,* and began to *elevate the head of the bed, provide oxygen by nasal cannula, and auscultate breath sounds.* The nurse called the physician and received an order for IV furosemide. As a result of the nurse's actions the client *experienced diuresis and decreased work of breathing and had an O_2 saturation of 93%.*

Box 6–5.
Nuts and Bolts Exercise

Right Congestive Heart Failure

Once upon a time there was a *78-year-old woman* who had *chronic right ventricular heart failure* and was *brought to the Emergency Department for treatment* by her *85-year-old husband.* The nurse assessed the client and determined that she had *hepatomegaly, pedal edema scored at +4, related pain in the extremities, hypertension (BP 160/106 mm Hg), jugular vein distention, and a weight gain of 4 kg in the last 2 weeks.* The nurse began to *arrange the client in the position of comfort.* The nurse called the physician, who examined the client and ordered IV furosemide. As a result of the nurse's actions the client *experienced diuresis, the pedal edema decreased to +2, and her weight decreased 1 kg.*

Ideas for Use

- Use this exercise as the subject of a **Clinical Quick Write** or an **E-mail Exercise.** You can give out the forms and let the students pick the scenarios, or you can have them complete the assignment on a client you've selected.
- Ask students to compose the initial sentence for a **Nuts and Bolts** exercise and then switch papers in class so they can complete a classmate's story.

Box 6–6.
Nuts and Bolts Exercise

Hyperglycemia

Once upon a time there was *an 8-year-old boy* who had *type 1 diabetes mellitus* and was brought to the pediatric Emergency Department for evaluation and treatment. The nurse assessed the client and determined that *he* had *dry skin and fruity-smelling breath, was thirsty, complained of frequently needing to "pee," was disoriented, and felt nauseated. The client voided, and the nurse found large ketones in his urine. The nurse assessed the blood sugar, found it to be 450 mg/dL,* and began to *set up an IV for hydration and prepare to administer ordered insulin.* As a result of the nurse's actions the client *became more lucid, his urine tested for small ketones, his blood sugar decreased to 300 mg/dL, and he stated that he felt better.*

Box 6–7.
Nuts and Bolts Exercise

Hypoglycemia

Once upon a time there was *an 8-year-old boy* who had *type 1 diabetes mellitus* and was brought to the pediatric Emergency Department for evaluation and treatment. The nurse assessed the client and determined that *he* had *a decreased level of consciousness and visual disturbances and was sweaty. The client complained of hunger, a headache, and "shakiness." The nurse checked his blood sugar level, found it to be 45 mg/dL,* and gave the client *4 oz of juice (15 gm carbohydrate). After 15 minutes the nurse rechecked the blood sugar and found it to be 55 mg/dL. The 15 gm of glucose was repeated.* As a result of the nurse's action, *15 minutes later the client's blood sugar was 95 mg/dL. The nurse provided a snack with fat and protein.*

- Use **Think-Pair-Share** to encourage discussion.
- **Nuts and Bolts** is especially valuable for discriminating between difficult concepts. This strategy requires critical thinking skills: identifying the first nursing action and the highest nursing priority, and understanding the gravity of the client's signs and symptoms.
- This is a good strategy for helping students differentiate the subtle differences between two similar conditions. It works for mental

health disorders (e.g., borderline personality and bipolar disorders) and medical-surgical conditions (e.g., arterial and venous peripheral vascular disorders). You can use it to differentiate conditions within specialties (e.g., bacterial versus viral meningitis, abruptio placentae versus placenta previa, bone conduction versus nerve conduction hearing loss).

- Have students split into groups and reach a consensus on how to fill in the **Nuts and Bolts** blanks.

Teaching Tools

General Description   The main premise of this strategy is that we often undervalue the teaching tools we use to educate clients. These tools can be easily adapted for teaching both students and new or experienced nurses. **Teaching Tools** also reminds nurses to see clients as knowledgeable health-care partners and to remain current about what clients need to know.

Preparation and Equipment   You'll need to consider your own methods of educating clients about disease, treatment, diagnostic testing, medications, symptom management, and activities of daily living. Look in books and other resources on client education, general nursing, community health, and self-care; your class may well find them useful. Use diagnosis- or condition-appropriate teaching resources and clarify the level of information a client should receive. Students are often shocked at the amount and technical nature of client education materials. The role of the nurse in client education takes on new meaning for them.

Example of the Strategy at Work   I used the following tool in a lesson on client education. It not only emphasizes the importance of assessing the client's learning style, but reminds students to assess their own as well. The following example is inspired by a learner assessment recommended by Hunt.[4] This kind of **Teaching Tool** also works as an icebreaker and as a way to assess learning styles in your class.

Assessing the Learner
Brain Dominance

1. Likes words, numbers, letters, parts, sequential order, linear thought, language; is detail-oriented and organized (left-brained, analytical learner)
2. Likes images, patterns, entirety, simultaneous actions, music; is nonverbal, creative, intuitive, spontaneous, and graphics-oriented (right-brained, global learner)

Learning Modalities

1. Prefers verbal instruction; remembers names, not faces; is distracted by noise; enjoys music; likes answering machines (auditory learner)
2. Remembers faces, not names; has a vivid imagination; thinks in pictures; uses colors; likes postcards (visual learner)
3. Learns by doing and touching; remembers what was done; is impulsive; loves games (kinesthetic learner)

Favorite Learning Activities

Visual: Television, reading, videos, handouts, flipcharts, signs, writing

Auditory: Books on tape, tapes, music, radio, conversation, listening to steps

Kinesthetic: Games, simulations, group activities, role playing, demonstration

Ideas for Use:

*   Lead a class discussion on the reading level and comprehensibility of client education material. Ask students to brainstorm obstacles and solutions (Box 6–8).
*   Reinforce in every class the complexity of material nurses need to learn. Ask students to consider the impact of that complexity on the average client and family.
*   Many nursing textbooks include client education materials. Students, and nurses new to a condition or treatment, can use those **Teaching Tools** to educate themselves as well as clients.
*   Ask students to develop short client education materials based on a reading level. Computer programs, books, and word-processing software can be helpful in calculating reading levels.
*   In an elective class on diabetes, I was able to acquire the education packet for newly diagnosed clients with type 1 diabetes. This became the primary textbook for the course. It provided an excellent resource for both the material itself and the information a client with this condition would need.
*   Use the Internet to access patient education tools that may prove invaluable for nursing students and

Box 6–8.
Brainstorming Session

What do you do when a client:

*   Doesn't read?
*   Reads at a third-grade level?
*   Doesn't speak or read English?
*   Is visually impaired?

nurse orientees. Again, assist new nurses in the development of critiquing skills to ensure sound, evidence-based information.

- Experienced nurses can review client education materials provided by agencies. Ask them to evaluate the materials for their currency and usefulness in nursing orientation. This technique teaches both content and the policies and procedures of the agency.
- Sign on to Web-based listservs within the specialty and encourage the sharing of education materials. Use these materials in the clinical area to teach the value of sharing in this capacity.
- Assign students or orientees to research client education materials for a specific illness or client need. Have students present these to each other in a **Student-led Seminar.**

Day in the Life of a Client with . . .

General Description   This is a great strategy. It was suggested to me by a class participant. Each student selects a disease and spends one day "living the life" of a client with that condition. The students research the illness, consider its impact on the client throughout the day, and then plan how to live that life in conjunction with daily routine. Then comes the hard part: they actually simulate living with the illness. The students then compose a journal, much like an **Ah-hah Journal,** to summarize their experiences and reflect on the lessons learned.

Preparation and Equipment   In an academic setting, you need to assign conditions for students to simulate. You also need to design the assignment and evaluation methods. In the practice setting, use **Day in the Life of a Client with . . .** during orientation to teach new employees about predominant diagnoses or client conditions.

Example of the Strategy at Work   An instructor assigned each member of the clinical group to a different illness. In this exercise, students explored and experienced such diagnoses as type 1 diabetes mellitus, heart block with a pacemaker, chronic obstructive pulmonary disease on oxygen therapy, end-stage renal disease on dialysis, liver failure requiring a paracentesis, inoperable cataracts with significant visual impairment, cystic fibrosis requiring chest percussion and postural drainage, cerebrovascular accident sequelae with aphasia, breast cancer postmastectomy and on chemotherapy, spinal cord injury with paralysis, and congestive heart failure with significant activity intolerance.

Students considered the equipment needed, the dietary restrictions, the symptoms and limitation imposed by the illness, and activities of daily living. Then they worked out how to survive with the limitations and accomplish the instrumental activities of daily living (e.g., shopping, home maintenance and cleaning, banking).

Ideas for Use

- Students may do this exercise in pairs. One participant "lives the disease"; the other records challenges and issues and provides assistance as needed.
- **Day in the Life of a Client with . . .** is a great empathy-building exercise. It may be carried out as elaborately or as simply as class objectives require.
- In practice settings this strategy can be more cognitive. Novice nurses or nurses new to a setting can conjecture what it would be like to live a **Day in the Life of a Client with . . .**
- Many nursing diagnoses may be adapted to this strategy.
- Ask students to keep a log of activities throughout the day, including meals eaten, obstacles encountered, and experiences with symptoms, such as shortness of breath or fatigue.
- Each assigned condition should have a significant physical limitation. The student should experience inconvenience, potential pain, diet and activity restrictions, or a change in daily routine.
- This strategy introduces students to the different skills and equipment needed to care for their diagnosis. Skills may include principles of oxygen therapy, insulin administration, chest therapy, and others.
- Have students **Write to Learn** by doing a reaction paper based on preliminary research and personal experience.
- **Day in the Life of a Client with . . .** may be done in discussion groups, small classes, orientation groups, and clinical groups.
- Students can report their findings to other students in **One-Minute Classes** or **Grand Rounds.**
- Students can use **Ah-hah Journals** to document their experience.
- A quick rendition of this exercise has students or new nurses navigate the campus or agency in a wheelchair. This experience offers poignant insights. Students encounter firsthand the challenges of wheelchair dependence and of accommodations that are theoretically wheelchair appropriate, yet remain an obstacle for many clients.

Invented Dialogues

General Description   Nursing students and novice nurses must master the challenge of communicating and interacting outside their comfort zone.

Nurses have the privilege of quick entry into their clients' private lives, often being privy to intimate details. New nurses may not be equipped to deal with such candor, nor do they have the tools to respond therapeutically.

In this strategy, students respond to statements designed by the instructor. The responses should be appropriate, feasible, and comfortable for both participants in the conversation. **Invented Dialogues** are based on the class objectives and may be used in a variety of ways.

Preparation and Equipment   Clinical practice provides you with the potential statements to begin forming this exercise. Think about times when clients have confessed personal facts to you and you were either at a loss for words or needed to formulate an appropriate response quickly. These are the types of statements that make great conversation starters for **Invented Dialogues.** Think about times in the clinical area when students appeared to be stymied by a client's comment or question and how they should, or could, have responded.

Example of the Strategy at Work   I've used this strategy in a class on sex and sexuality. The idea of responding to clients' comments about sexuality made the students uncomfortable; **Invented Dialogues** gave them a chance to practice. Because this topic was so sensitive for some participants, I showed the statements on the screen, read each aloud, and paused to let the students consider their personal responses. Then I asked each student to formulate one response and send it to me as an **E-mail Exercise.** Here are some of the statements and questions used in that class:

- "I told the doctor I don't take Viagra but I really do."
- "I'm afraid my husband doesn't love me since my mastectomy."
- "I'd like to take you out to dinner once I get out of the hospital."
- "Will the diabetes prevent me from having an erection?"
- "I don't take my medicine because I heard it causes impotence."
- "I don't want to wear condoms when I have sex."
- "I'm a homosexual but I don't want anyone at the hospital to know."

You can use **Invented Dialogues** in class discussion, with class members suggesting responses. I also used this strategy, with statements from students instead of clients, to teach nurse educators about creative teaching strategies. Here are the statements I used to stimulate responses during our class discussion:

- "I had to cheat on the assignment; I ran out of time."
- "I didn't have time to give the bath because I needed to look up my medications today in clinical. I didn't look up all my meds last night because I didn't have time."

- "My client says he doesn't want to get out of bed and the MD wants him to walk three times a day."
- "The nurse yesterday said meds can be 1-hour late. The nurse today said only one-half hour. Who do I believe?"
- "Just tell me what's on the test."
- " Why do I have to participate? I'd rather just listen."
- "I can't come to class; I have to work."
- "I don't like to write things on a calendar."

Ideas for Use

- In a large classroom, you can show the statements as a PowerPoint slide and ask for immediate responses.
- This strategy can be used as a **Think-Pair-Share.** Student pairs develop responses to the statements and discuss how the client might react. This method highlights the circular nature of communication and the impact of a nurse's answer on a client's attitude and behavior.
- **Invented Dialogues** are generally more comfortable than more elaborate role-play exercises. Its brevity keeps the discussion from becoming more detailed and perhaps uncomfortable.
- For larger classes or to provide anonymity, you can combine this strategy with **Clinical Quick Writes, E-mail Exercises,** and **Admit Tickets.**
- Use class objectives to develop statements, especially for sensitive subjects such as spirituality, sexuality, high-risk behaviors, and legal or ethical conflicts.
- **Invented Dialogues** are great for practicing responses in clinical situations. Comments from clients may include:
  - "I don't want to take a bath today."
  - "I don't want a student nurse."
  - "I haven't had any pain meds since yesterday. I'm sorry the nurse told you I did, but I haven't had any."
  - "I don't want to quit smoking; why should I?"
  - "I don't know how to read."
  - "I don't understand the surgery I'm having today."
  - "I don't take my medicine because it's too expensive."
  - "I take herbs with my medicine but haven't told my doctor."
  - "I don't want to be in this research study anymore."
  - "I feel like I have no reason for living."
  - "My dad hit me really hard last night and I'm not allowed to tell anyone."

This last statement touches on the topic of the nurse's role in an abusive situation and how it may depend on the age of the client.

- The following situation can help to clarify a nurse's role when a fellow nurse is impaired: A nurse colleague says to you, "I need to sign out some narcotics, so don't ask any questions."
- The following example may be used in teaching isolation precautions: Ask the class for their response if a nurse says, "You don't need to use all these isolation procedures. I've been a nurse a long time and I've never caught anything."

Guided Discussion Groups

General Description   Discussion groups can be difficult to maintain. They're especially vulnerable at the beginning or end of the semester, at other busy times, in summer, and near holidays. At these times instructors need strategies that are objective driven and valuable, but also fun and a change of pace from the normal classroom routine. A **Guided Discussion Group** can help. When traditional teaching methods become too mundane, the instructor can entertain the group with creative exercises that also reflect their learning needs.

Preparation and Equipment   This strategy may take a little more work than usual. It's actually a combination of several creative strategies woven into a single learning session.

Example of the Strategy at Work   **Guided Discussion Groups** have been effective in teaching such concepts as wellness and the nurse's role in stress management. Used in both academic and clinical settings, the following exercises focus on nurses' need to manage their own stress while fostering stress management strategies in their clients.

Are You Stress Resistant?
We begin with this assessment to set the stage for continued discussion:

I. This is a quick measure of your ability to resist stress! Score 0 if the statement is not true for you; 1 if it's usually not true; 2 if it's somewhat true; and 3 if it definitely is true.

1. _____ When I work hard it makes a difference.
2. _____ Getting out of bed in the morning is easy for me.
3. _____ I have the freedom I want and need.
4. _____ At times I have sacrificed for an exciting opportunity.
5. _____ Sticking to my routine is not important to me.
6. _____ I vote because I think it makes a difference.

7. _____ I make my own lucky breaks.
8. _____ I agree with the goals of my boss, company, school, or family.
9. _____ I've been lucky in love because I try to be a loving person.
10. _____ I believe I get what I give but I don't keep score.
11. _____ It is important for me to try new things.
12. _____ Free time is a gift I really enjoy.
13. _____ I work hard and I'm paid fairly.
14. _____ My family is a great pleasure to me.
15. _____ I speak up for what I believe in.

SCORING:

Add your scores for questions 1, 6, 7, 9, and 13. This is your stress management score. The higher it is, the more control you feel you have over your own life. The better able you are to manage your own stress.

TOTAL: _____

Add your scores for questions 2, 3, 8, 10, and 14. This is your commitment score. The higher it is, the more committed you are to enhancing and enjoying your life.

TOTAL: _____

Add your scores for questions 4, 5, 11, 12, and 15. This is your risk score. The higher it is, the more willing you are to take risks.

TOTAL: _____

Add the three scores together. This is your stress resistance score:

OVERALL TOTAL: _____

If you score 35 or more: Congratulations, you are very resistant to stress and your attitudes help you.

If you score 27–34: You are somewhat stress resistant but could be more so. Look at each item and choose a few to work on.

If you score 18–27: You need to look at your habits and attitudes and improve your resistance to stress. Select one area to improve each month.

If your score is less than 18: If stress gets serious you could be in trouble—take time now to change your habits and attitudes.

Happy stress resisting!

II. Following that assessment, we discuss common stressors in a lecture-discussion format in which I write down the stressors on a flipchart or blackboard.

III. After this activity, students are asked to discuss the following questions in **Group.**

THOUGHT:

1. How do you know when you're stressed? What physical and emotional signals let you know you're stressed?
2. How do you generally manage your stress? Do those strategies work?
3. What interventions would you like to employ to more effectively deal with stress?
4. What lifestyle habits keep you from being stress resistant? What lifestyle habits enhance your stress resistance?
5. What is the role of the nurse in assisting clients to recognize stress and become stress resistant?

IV. The final activity has students frame stress management in terms of the nurse's role. Students write a **One-Minute Care Plan** for a partner based on a brief **Think-Pair-Share** about stress assessment and management. Each student is asked to use the nursing diagnosis of *Ineffective individual coping related to* _____ *as evidenced by* _____ . Each student develops one long-term goal, two short-term goals, and two interventions for each short-term goal. These **One-Minute Care Plans** should be individualized for the client using the data collected in the previous conversations.

Ideas for Use

- Use a **Guided Discussion Group** when addressing controversial or difficult issues. Nursing ethics, values clarification, assertiveness skills, professional issues, and therapeutic client relationships may all require more than lecture and discussion. As I've shown, this strategy combines several different strategies in a concerted learning package. This approach may prove more effective and enjoyable than one strategy used alone.

- One of the greatest assets of **Guided Discussion Groups** is the repetition of material in several formats. Repetition is a form of mental aerobics, in which the mind practices material and exercises the brain.

- Combine several strategies with **Guided Discussion Groups** to yield the best results: **Think-Pair-Share, Admit Ticket, Same**

Information, Critical Thinking Exercises, and others can augment the learning and the fun.

- The final **One-Minute Care Plan** may be handed in at the end of class, written and handed in later, or submitted electronically as an **E-mail Exercise.**
- **Guided Discussion Groups** may be adapted to any course content. You'll meet class objectives simply by collecting several exercises and strategies and developing a schedule for their use.

Out of the Hat

General Description   In this strategy, the instructor creates a pool of topics to be discussed or evaluated. Students then select one or more topics **Out of the Hat** and are asked to demonstrate understanding and competency in those areas. This is a common testing strategy when a lot of material must be assessed in a limited amount of time; examples include physical assessment and basic nursing skills. Alternatively, students can create a **One-Minute Class, Student-led Seminar,** or **Ah-hah Journal** based on the selected topic.

Preparation and Equipment   The equipment you'll need depends on the skills to be tested. You can use this strategy to test psychomotor skills. Ask students to assemble the supplies needed for the task they've just pulled **Out of the Hat.**

Example of the Strategy at Work   Traditionally, this strategy has been used to assess psychomotor competency. Health assessment courses teach skills sequentially. You can use **Out of the Hat** to test assessment of neurological, respiratory, cardiac, integumentary, gastrointestinal, and other systems. Students come prepared to be tested on any system. They don't know which one they'll be tested on until they pick it **Out of the Hat.**

Out of the Hat also works for testing out fundamental skills. We came up with a Total Care Test Out to test basic skills. Students practiced hygiene, body mechanics, assessing vital signs, making beds, moving clients, and various other basic skills throughout the semester.

In the Total Care Test Out, pairs of students demonstrated handwashing, vital signs, giving a bed bath, brushing a client's teeth, and making an occupied bed. Then they picked two other skills **Out of the Hat.** These included putting a client on a bedpan, applying wrist restraints, teaching walker or crutch walking, stretcher transfer, and shaving. They also selected a position (supine, prone, Fowler's, Sims', lateral) **Out of the Hat.** This strategy cut down on the time needed to test each student while ensuring that each one had prepared every skill.

Ideas for Use

- **Out of the Hat** allows you to evaluate competency in any psychomotor skill.
- This strategy is appropriate for discussion groups, clinical groups, or small groups in classes with a psychomotor component.
- **Out of the Hat** allows students to demonstrate their knowledge of a topic orally. Evaluate content mastery by having students pick a class concept or topic **Out of the Hat** and explain it to classmates.
- Let students pick out one of the topics for that day's class. Each **Out of the Hat** topic is then discussed at length. Students may also pick out discussion questions and potential issues related to a class topic. You're available to clarify issues, but the students lead the discussion.
- For orientation groups and nurses accomplishing mandatory requirements, **Out of the Hat** makes a good alternative to written post-tests. Each nurse picks a topic **Out of the Hat** and answers orally or does a **Clinical Quick Write.** Staff development instructors can use checklists to document these demonstrations.
- **Out of the Hat** may be used for part or all of a class session. It can add flavor to another exercise: students pick the topic for an **In-class Debate,** a partner for an icebreaker or **Think-Pair-Share,** or a role in a **Teaching Trio.**
- Students may pick topics for oral presentations **Out of the Hat.**

Legal Cheat Sheets

General Description   Cheating is a funny thing. If students spent as much time studying as they did preparing eloquent cheat sheets, their test performance would excel. **Legal Cheat Sheets** let students select priority points in any class and develop them into study sheets with the instructor's help. These **Legal Cheat Sheets** become flash cards for studying material, focusing on most important content, and setting priorities among key issues.

Legal Cheat Sheets work well with material that's often memorized, such as lab values, norms, difficult concepts, and numerical data. This strategy moves such information from one category to another: "need to remember" becomes "need to know where to find it." Students find more freedom to think critically and develop prioritization and decision-making skills. Less encumbered with the need to memorize, they can look beyond the facts to the potential contexts that surround those facts and influence nursing practice.

Preparation and Equipment   Your only preparation for this strategy is to guide students in developing personal **Legal Cheat Sheets** for later use. You can help by suggesting a format for the sheets. In addition, you can create a classroom environment in which **Legal Cheat Sheets** are an accepted aid to learning, studying, and evaluation.

Example of the Strategy at Work   Students are encouraged to use **Legal Cheat Sheets** as study guides for test preparation. Often they spend a significant amount of time selecting which material should go on the sheet. This prioritization process encourages students to select and study material that's integral to the test or the course. After the initial reading and class preparation, students revisit the material while selecting integral information, formatting the cheat sheet, writing information in the cheat sheet, reviewing, and finally while studying for the test. This is a good example of the mental aerobics—the repetition—so important in learning. This strategy works regardless of learning style.

Ideas for Use

- Allow students to bring **Legal Cheat Sheets** to examinations. They'll feel more at liberty to use critical thinking and decision-making skills rather than focusing only on memorization. This method replicates many clinical practice settings in which memorization is no longer emphasized. Standard practice emphasizes the ability to find accurate information quickly, especially in emergency situations.
- Use this strategy as a means to study and review for final examinations. A semester's worth of **Legal Cheat Sheets** provides a compendium of review materials. Keeping up with **Legal Cheat Sheets** throughout the semester or the course creates a study guide for comprehensive final examinations.
- Encourage students to work in pairs, trios, or groups to enhance their **Legal Cheat Sheets.**
- **Quizzes, Student-led Seminars, Gaming,** and **E-mail Exercises** may all be combined with **Legal Cheat Sheets** to add to their educational value.
- Students may be encouraged to share their **Legal Cheat Sheets** through **Online Discussion Groups** or in **Group Thought.** Students can rotate responsibility for compiling **Legal Cheat Sheets** in different subjects.
- Students can help each other by sharing their **Legal Cheat Sheets** during study groups and review sessions.
- Use **Legal Cheat Sheets** to summarize and reinforce key material from slides and class notes.

Mock Trials

General Description   **Mock Trials** serve two purposes. They address the legal and ethical conflicts inherent in nursing and health care, and provide practice in organizing and delivering a presentation. This presentation mimics a courtroom trial.

Preparation and Equipment   Because this strategy requires a lot of work from students, it's probably most effective in the academic setting. You will need to determine the evaluation method for the assignment.

Example of the Strategy at Work   In a continuing education program an attorney was asked to present the legal aspects of nursing documentation. Knowing that this could be a dry issue, she created a **Mock Trial** about the hazards of poor documentation. Volunteers from the audience were solicited in advance to take roles and given mini-scripts to follow.

The attorney then created a courtroom vignette. A nurse on the witness stand was asked to relate events of several years ago that had ended in a client's death. The nurse was provided with the documentation surrounding the incident. Her testimony exposed major lapses such as illegibility, documentation once per shift, undocumented care, spelling errors, the use of correction fluid, and other poor practices. The speaker masterfully met all the class objectives in 1 hour and had the rapt attention of the class the entire time.

Ideas for Use

- A **Mock Trial** may be incorporated into a continuing education program as an entertaining way to address a legal issue or conflict.
- **Mock Trials** are effective ways to reinforce the need for careful documentation at all levels of nursing.
- Agency ethical rounds can use a **Mock Trial** as a platform to discuss the needs and roles of the multidisciplinary team in ethically difficult circumstances.
- Have students select a legal issue and act as a group to establish roles and scripts. Group members may serve as defendants, lawyers, plaintiffs, a judge, witnesses, and jury members.
- Plan a discussion group in which the **Mock Trial** is an impromptu event, allowing students to take roles and wade their way through the dialogue.
- In a more formal **Mock Trial,** you can assign roles and have brief scripts written out on index cards. Students may be encouraged to ad lib as necessary.
- **Mock Trials** may be used in a research class to help teach the rights of human subjects. These include autonomy, informed

consent, the risk-to-benefit ratio, and beneficence. You develop a case representing an infringement of these rights, the **Mock Trial** follows, and the class discusses the issue. Other concepts may include failure to disclose risks, participation under duress or coercion, or unethical research practices.

- Use a **Mock Trial** to approach several legal issues, such as negligence, malpractice, false imprisonment, and fraud.
- Use case law to develop a realistic subject for the **Mock Trial.**
- As in a debate, students should be evaluated on their level of research, knowledge of the topic, ability to present their case within their role, and contribution to the group.
- A small group may present the **Mock Trial** for extra credit. Other students may write their reactions as an **E-mail Exercise** or a variant on the **Clinical Quick Write.**
- Students may witness the **Mock Trial** and then be asked to apply their knowledge by answering questions related to a different case study.
- Encourage groups to share the preparation and dialogue evenly. Students can share roles and assist each other in presenting extensive material.
- Have an attorney visit the class to discuss major legal concepts and then use them in the **Mock Trial.**
- Use the **Mock Trial** as a way to reinforce documentation skills in the clinical area. After students complete the **Documentation Case Study,** create a **Mock Trial** scenario. Ask students to go back and look at the care they "delivered" in the case and use their documentation to reconstruct that care. Discuss gaps or discrepancies that could be misinterpreted or are difficult to evaluate. Emphasize that it's this type of documentation issue that creates legal conflicts. What a great way to reinforce accurate and comprehensive documentation!

Learning Carts

General Description   This strategy works the way it sounds: you place your educational materials on a cart and take it to your students. This cart conveys the message "I am here to teach you" and signals that learning is the order of the day. **Learning Carts** allow instructors to bring in all the necessary equipment and to move the learning location as needed.

Preparation and Equipment   Of course, this strategy requires a cart—or a box, carrying case, or whatever allows you to transport teaching materials easily. The size will depend on what you plan to transport.

Some **Learning Carts** include a laptop computer and a DVD player, a slide projector, or an overhead projector. A blank wall on which to project images eliminates the need for a screen. Other equipment depends on the skills or material being taught and on the needs of the instructor. You could bring handouts, games, puzzles, prizes, models, pre- and post-tests, audiovisual equipment, supplies for skills, other materials, and snacks and beverages (these always attract learners).

Example of the Strategy at Work   **Learning Carts** are most effective in staff development and agency settings, where unit-to-unit education meets the needs of busy staff nurses. This strategy communicates your desire to teach and your appreciation of the factors that often keep nurses from participating in educational programs. **Learning Carts** also keep you ready for repeated teaching sessions. You just take the cart and go! Agencies have used this strategy to teach staff about a new piece of equipment or a hospital-wide policy change, to help them meet mandatory requirements, to prepare for an accreditation survey, and to assess the competency of nurses in or just ending their orientation.

In academic settings, in which lab or hospital space is at a premium, **Learning Carts** can bring the setting to the students rather than vice versa. Sometimes labs become so crowded that it's difficult for every student to see a demonstration. A colleague of mine wheels a hospital bed into a traditional classroom to teach moving the client in bed and positioning. She packs a **Learning Cart** with needed supplies, a DVD demonstrating the skills, a short pre- and post-test, and supplies (e.g., draw sheets, pillows, towels). The entire class sees the demonstration at once, and each student has a clear view of the procedure. Students then go to the lab to practice the skills on their own.

Ideas for Use

- Come up with your own **Learning Cart** contents and use them consistently for every class you teach.
- Have students or orientees develop a seminar or presentation and set up their own **Learning Cart.** Role model the use of a **Learning Cart** during orientation.
- Keep **Learning Cart** teaching sessions short and to the point. Leave handouts or graded post-tests to reinforce the sessions.
- Allow students to work in pairs, trios, or groups to create a **Learning Cart.**
- Do a procedure review by having clinical groups work in pairs and develop a **Learning Cart.** Encourage them to set up an **Active Reading Conference** to review the procedural protocol and the necessary equipment and supplies needed for the procedure. Have them

use active teaching strategies to involve the entire group. Let students pick the skill to be discussed **Out of the Hat.** Students may research the skill and use **Clinical Area Questioning** or **Bring on the Evidence** to determine the evidence base for the skill or procedure.

- Make sure you hand out prizes or small gifts as a way to thank learners and student teachers for their time.
- Use a variety of **Case Studies** along with equipment from the **Learning Cart** to address a learning topic.
- When the teaching materials allow, use bins or boxes to carry class supplies from one area to another. Let the bin be the signal that learning is about to occur for units, satellite clinics, or during a clinical rotation!

Pass the Stick

General Description   This quick strategy helps to control a discussion group. Simply, the stick is passed around the group, and whoever has the stick has the floor.

Preparation and Equipment   You guessed it—you need a stick! You'll also need to set ground rules for its use. Parameters may include timing, which way to pass it, the need to observe the rules, and other details specific to the exercise.

Example of the Strategy at Work   I learned this strategy from a colleague who has taught first grade for a long time. Simple though it is, it meets two important goals. Discussion groups always have some participants who rarely contribute and others who monopolize the conversation. The stick ensures that those who don't generally talk are given that opportunity and that those who talk excessively have some limits on their participation. The stick provides parameters for all group members—it allows all members to participate. Only those with the stick may talk and you don't talk unless you have it.

Ideas for Use

- You can use a toy magic wand instead of a stick. You could also use a baton—hence the term "pass the baton."
- This strategy is an effective way to get everyone in a group to talk. In a discussion of conflicts or sensitive issues, some group members may not disclose their thoughts readily. **Pass the Stick** requires they participate at least to some small extent.
- **Pass the Stick** may be used with **Imagine** or **Remember When, Reality Check, Mock Trials, In-class Debates,** or **Case Studies** to ensure contributions and equal sharing.

- In a clinical group, **Pass the Stick** may be used to facilitate **Grand Rounds, V-8 Conferences, Learning from Each Other,** and other post-conference topics.
- **Pass the Stick** may be used to assess or test the class. You can **Pass the Stick** around the group to ask questions, pose issues, or test skills.

Put It All Together

General Description   **Put It All Together** gives students an opportunity to synthesize material. Students pick a condition or a diagnosis (medical or nursing) that interests them. Alternatively, they may pick a client they've cared for in clinical rotation. Then they augment their past experience or clinical knowledge with continued research in the chosen area. This strategy thoroughly investigates many aspects of nursing or of a particular client. **Put It All Together** is a good summative assignment for a clinical or senior-level course. Pared down and used at the end of an agency orientation, it can reinforce knowledge of conditions seen frequently in that facility.

Preparation and Equipment   You'll need to come up with the criteria for this strategy. When the exercise involves a particular client, the following topics should be addressed:

- Description of the medical or nursing diagnosis
- Client demographics
- Pathophysiology of the condition
- Physical signs and symptoms
- Assessments
- Diagnostic, lab, and medical imaging data
- Client history and risk factors
- Nursing care—specific to the condition (may include client goals and nursing strategies)
- Nursing care—general (may include client goals and nursing strategies)
- Nutrition and diet therapy
- Medical treatment: medications, hydration, treatments, procedures, surgeries
- Potential complications—both rare and common ones and associated nursing monitoring
- Appropriate precautions (e.g., bleeding, aspiration, seizure, neutropenia, fall)
- Client teaching, discharge, family teaching
- Psychoemotional issues

In certain conditions, other topics may need to be addressed.

Once you decide which information needs to be included, you can choose a variety of formats for this exercise. Possibilities include a conference or seminar, a poster or chart, a report, a nursing care plan, a client profile, and a discussion group. These are only some of the ways your students can show their ability to **Put It All Together.**

Example of the Strategy at Work   This strategy allows students in discussion groups to develop a capstone assignment at the end of a course. Using the information previously listed, each of my students created a database, developed and handed out a one-page nursing care plan, and presented a 10-minute seminar in class. It's critical to tell the class that this assignment is meant to **Put It All Together.** After sifting through a wealth of information, students must establish priorities before they can condense it all into a 10-minute presentation.

In this exercise, I place a lot of emphasis on laboratory diagnostics. Although students understand the lab abnormalities associated with a diagnosis, they don't always grasp their dynamic nature. A change in lab values means a change in the client's status, and the nurse has a vital role in monitoring these values.

My students have presented such topics as pancreatitis, hepatitis, spinal cord injury, different types of cancer, chronic obstructive pulmonary disease, asthma, diabetes, epilepsy, and head injury. These presentations often lead to interesting discussions about which aspects of care are common and which differ according to condition.

Ideas for Use

- Students may select a client who interests them or one they cared for in a clinical rotation. Alternatively, you can assign a client whose condition ties in with class objectives.
- You can establish guidelines at your discretion. For example, you can gear the assignment toward clinical specialty, course needs, student level, available time, and percentage of the course grade.
- In orientation groups, each participant can present a client and a brief care plan for that client. A new nurse can present a selected client, cared for during orientation, whose condition is commonly encountered on the nursing unit.
- Combine this strategy with **Grand Rounds** or **Learning from Each Other.** Students can present the highlights of a case to the group and hand in the comprehensive report.
- Ask students to consider **What's the Big Deal?** and the **Muddiest Part** when selecting information to present to their colleagues.

- Allow students some creativity with this assignment. **Group Concept Mapping, Dress-up or Skits,** and other creative exercises can enhance their presentation.
- Use a **One-Minute Care Plan** to establish nursing priorities and allow students to focus on nursing care.
- **Put It All Together** cultivates presentation skills and assertiveness in addition to building students' knowledge base and appreciation of their role in client care (Herrman[2]).
- **Put It All Together** can form the structure for an entire course. Students use readings and course objectives to prepare for class. Rotating presentations feature different prototype conditions at each class session. Finally, the instructor rounds out the information in a summary discussion. In this form, **Put It All Together** develops priority-setting skills and confers many of the same benefits as **Learning from Each Other.**

FYI—Classroom Questioning

General Description   Here, **Classroom Questioning** is the strategy; **FYI** (For Your Information) is the purpose. It's important to note that "Your" refers to both instructors and students at any educational level.

FYI—Classroom Questioning is an effective way for learners to assess their own level of knowledge, find out if they're on track, determine whether their knowledge base can meet course objectives, or clarify areas of confusion. Instructors can find many uses for **Classroom Questioning** (Box 6–9).

Preparation and Equipment   Little preparation is required. **FYI—Classroom Questioning** is more a teaching philosophy than a distinct strategy. You may find yourself using it in every class to assess your

---

Box 6–9.
FYI—Classroom Questioning

Learn About Your Class
- What do they know?
- Are they well prepared for class?
- Are they ready for the next topic?
- Do they need a pep talk to get them going?
- Do you need to revisit a topic?
- Should you change any assignments or due dates?

students and create a reciprocal atmosphere. You should consider potential questions while preparing your class.

Example of the Strategy at Work   Classroom questioning can be tough. Students may come unprepared or busy themselves with note taking or other activities. They'll ask you to repeat your content, spell a word, or clarify a simple concept. This type of questioning is not what **FYI—Classroom Questioning** refers to. In this strategy, students and instructors ask and answer questions that demonstrate, provoke, and encourage critical thinking.

Both instructors and students must learn to ask "good" questions. This type of questioning is usually on the application or evaluation level. Classroom and staff development instructors should consider reviewing and adapting objective multiple-choice questions before class. When I give a test on venous thrombosis and anticoagulants, I might include the following question:

1. A client you are caring for has thrombophlebitis. The client is receiving heparin. You instruct the client that the action of heparin is to:

   a. Prolong the clotting time.
   b. Decrease the clotting time.
   c. Dissolve the blood clot.
   d. Inhibit the bleeding time.

This question may be adapted to "What is the action of heparin?" This question and the resulting discussion are at the retention level. We then use the next question to generate continued discussion:

2. A client with a chronic deep vein thrombosis is ordered to receive warfarin (Coumadin) at bedtime every night. The client complains of indigestion and is given an antacid with meals and at bedtime. Which of the following client statements indicates a need for more teaching?

   a. "I take the medications together at night with a snack."
   b. "I need to stop the Coumadin 2 weeks before I go to the dentist."
   c. "I take the Coumadin every day and the antacid as needed."
   d. "I need to take my medications with water."

The following discussion may include such issues as bleeding precautions, discharge instructions for a client on anticoagulant therapy, and interactions with other medications. This classroom discussion has reached the application level. To take it a step further, you can ask students to apply information about the disorder to teaching, evaluation for complications, nursing implications, and other issues that foster critical thinking. You might ask some of the following questions:

- Your client complains of significant mouth bleeding. What do you do?
- Your client needs to have dental work. What recommendations do you have?
- Your client is switched to warfarin after heparin and tells you he eats spinach every day. What recommendations do you have for this client?
- You client notices dark red blood in his stool. What could this be? What actions are appropriate at this time?
- Anticoagulant therapy is ordered for your client after a cerebro-vascular accident. He tells you he doesn't take any medications and doesn't want to start now. How do you respond?

The key to this strategy is to stimulate thinking. The answers should be longer than the questions; fewer words are needed for the question than are needed to develop a complex and complete answer.

Ideas for Use

- You don't need to use written questions in this strategy. Just remember to pause every so often to question and be questioned by the class.
- Be supportive of questions in the classroom. Make sure students who ask questions receive positive reinforcement, such as "That's a great question," or "I meant to cover that, thanks for the reminder."
- While preparing the lecture or presentation, consider what questions you'll ask and where you'll place them. **Use the Star** in your notes and to reinforce key pieces of information from the lecture.
- Oermann[5] suggests the One-Minute Question and Answer. Difficult areas of content are examined through a short question-ing period. Both instructors and students form pairs or groups to consider potential answers, and a class discussion follows.
- **Classroom Questioning** should be reflected in tests. **Use the Star** to signify a study topic for students and a question area for the instructor.
- Watch for those quizzical looks in class. They're a sure sign that you've reached the **Muddiest Part** and that some points need clarification. Things are also getting muddy when students start shaking their writing hand or ask you to repeat something two or three times, or when you hear a murmur go through the crowd.

Be alert to signals that the class is off track and help them get back on. Trudging ahead only leads to frustration and an increased sense of "lostness."

- See **Clinical Questioning** to adapt questions for the more intimate setting of the clinical environment.
- Use **Pass the Stick** to encourage questions that both stimulate the questioner and set off a discourse within the class.
- Try to stimulate students who don't participate by asking, "Are there any questions from someone I don't often hear from?" Follow that with eye contact to give the quieter students license to participate in class.
- Pose questions whether or not you plan to discuss them during class time. Ask students to provide answers through **E-mail Exercises, Clinical Quick Writes,** or **Online Discussion Groups.** This method generates discussion and rewards class attendance. Give extra credit for the correct answers relating to that day's content.
- "Round robin" the room, asking questions of each student. Class participation and the level of preparation will certainly increase. However, this technique can discourage class attendance, so it should be used carefully. Never use it to embarrass students who can't answer their questions.
- Use **Gaming** to stimulate questioning. In a variant of the 20 Questions game, students ask 20 questions to try to identify an illness or condition. Twenty questions may include:
  - Do both men and women get the illness?
  - Is it contagious?
  - Is it painful?
  - Can it be treated with antibiotics?
  - Does it happen with mostly older clients?
  - Does it change the complete blood count?
  - Is it visible?
  - Is it treated with surgery?
  - Does it affect the lungs? Gastrointestinal tract? Nervous system?
  - Does it require involved nursing care?

  Question–Question, described by Schell,[6] explores a case scenario by having each student pose a question. Each question is answered with another question. Students rotate throughout the room, asking questions that answer the previous question, being careful not to repeat questions or to speak in statements. These questions uncover increasing levels of complexity about an illness or condition and foster discussion of nursing priorities. *Jeopardy* and other game shows can model ways to structure questions and foster questioning skills.

- Respond positively when a student asks or answers a question. It rewards students to hear, "Good question, let me see if I can answer that for you," or "As we discussed, your question brings up . . . ." Responses such as, "We already talked about that," or "That questions is off track from this class," discourage participation on a regular basis. Students who answer questions need the same respect. Rather than saying, "No, that's wrong," try "That is an interesting point, but let me clarify by saying . . ." or "Sometimes what you say may be true, but more often . . . " Of course, if a student's conclusions are truly wrong, they need to be corrected. Again, framing that correction in a polite way invites the student to participate in class again.

- Make sure you leave enough time for students to either answer or ask questions. Nursing instructors often feel pressured to fit lessons into the allotted time frame and may not feel free to allow a **Classroom Questioning** period. When we ask a question, we often pause for 1 or 2 seconds and then answer our own question. You should allow 30 seconds for students to construct an answer. Although that seems like an eternity, it's important to impress on the class that you truly want their answers and will wait patiently for them to assemble their thoughts.

- Use **FYI—Classroom Questioning** to create healthy competition among students in **Gaming** or just within class discussion. Encourage questioning through **Prizes.**

- Ask students to ask their questions as part of the **Admit Ticket** or Exit Ticket.

References

1. Lyman, F: Think Pair Share: An expanding teaching technique. MAA-CIE Cooperative News Vol. 1:1–2, 1987.
2. Herrman, J: The 60-second nurse educator: Creative strategies to inspire learning. Nursing Education Perspective 23(5):222–227, 2002.
3. Beitz, J: Concept mapping: Navigating the learning process. Nurse Educator 23(5):35–41, 1998.
4. Hunt, R: Introduction to community-based nursing. Lippincott Williams & Wilkins, Philadelphia, 2005.
5. Oermann, MH: Using active learning in lecture: Best of "both worlds." International Journal of Nursing Education Scholarship l(1):1–9, 2004.
6. Schell, K: Promoting student questioning. Nurse Educator 23(5):8–12, 1998.

Personal Journal Pages

Chapter 7

Strategies for Teaching Research

> *"Education is not the filling of a pail, but the lighting of a fire."* —William Butler Yeats

> *"The highest result of education is tolerance."* —Helen Keller

Challenges

- Students express fear and anxiety about learning concepts important to nursing research and evidence-based practice.
- Nursing research may be taught in basic nursing curricula as a stand-alone course or integrated into content.
- Students and nurses don't see the clinical application of nursing research concepts.
- Students and nurses don't generally like to learn about nursing research.
- Nursing research and evidence-based practice are integral concepts for practicing nurses and agency accrediting organizations.
- Students busy with clinical courses see nursing research as a "fluff" course rather than a tool for improving nursing care and client outcomes.
- Content tends to be abstract and difficult to understand. Terminology may be totally new to both students and practicing nurses. Complex statistics and data analysis procedures often present roadblocks for nurses trying to grasp research concepts.
- Nursing research concepts usually differ greatly from other nursing clinical content.
- Educators vary widely in their knowledge of quantitative and qualitative research methods.
- Practicing nurses may take the attitude that nursing research is a subject they "had" to learn in school, or they may claim they're old enough to have "missed it."

Our evidence-based teaching and practice should include nursing research. The challenge is to make it understandable, useful, clinically relevant, and interesting.

IDEAS

Market Research—Cookies, Candy, and the Research Process

General Description   Comparison study in the classroom leads students through the steps of the research process. This strategy may also be used to illustrate specific research concepts.

Preparation and Equipment   Put two objects in a zippered plastic bag for each student in the class. These objects must be comparable at some level.

Example of the Strategy at Work   To teach the research process, I distribute cookies or candy and caution the students not to eat until they're directed to do so. On the screen or board, I show the research process step by step (Box 7–1).

I've found it interesting to compare two kinds of chocolate chip cookies because so many comparisons are possible (number of chips per cookie, taste, size, price, texture). As a class we discuss each step and raise interesting questions:

- What is the problem we are trying to research?
- How would we design the study?
- What key words would we include in the literature review?
- What does the literature have to say about market research and this study?

Box 7–1.
Cookie Research

1. State the research question.
2. Define the purpose.
3. Review the literature.
4. Formulate a hypothesis; define variables.
5. Select the research design.
6. Select the population, sample, and setting.
7. Conduct a pilot study.
8. Collect the data.
9. Analyze the data.
10. Communicate conclusions and implications.

- Who is the sample?
- How many sample members do we need?

Eventually we move into more complex discussion:

- Is this class (sample) representative of the target population?
- If I coerced you into participating in this study, what rights would I violate and what threats would I expose you to?
- What are the threats to internal and external validity?
- Why do businesses perform market research?

The last question leads to a discussion of the needs that motivate nursing research.

Ideas for Use

- Students enjoy food. You can use candy, cookies, crackers, or any food small enough to carry around. In large classes, consider your time and expense.
- You can ask students to develop hypotheses or research questions based on this strategy.
- After the exercise, you can open a discussion about sampling, sample sizes, or random sampling versus random assignment.
- Use **Market Research** for an entire class; as a group, trio, or pair exercise; or as a story incorporated into lecture content.
- Student groups can report their results to the rest of the class.

How Do You Pick Your Shampoo?

General Description   In a large or small group, students can be asked about the decision-making process used to select a brand of any product. Using the steps of the research process, students correlate research, decision-making, and the nursing process.

Preparation and Equipment   No special equipment is required. Bringing pictures of the product will stimulate your students to think creatively.

Example of the Strategy at Work   I show a slide of a model with gorgeous hair and ask the students what criteria they use to select their personal shampoo. We discuss such variables as cost, recommendations by friends, availability in the shower, desire for certain hair qualities, store displays, custom, exposure to advertising and marketing, recommendations from authority figures, previous experience, supermarket versus hair salon accessibility, expert advice from a hair stylist, and more (Box 7–2). These considerations

Box 7–2.
Shampoo Research

What influenced you?
- It's cheap.
- My friend likes it.
- I can hang the bottle in the shower.
- It makes my hair silky.
- It looked so pretty in the store.
- I've always used it.
- I kept seeing the ads on TV.
- My neighbor used to work as a beautician, and she says it's great.
- I can pick it up at the supermarket.
- My hair stylist likes his own special kind.

echo the "ways of knowing" that often guide nursing practice.

When we've exhausted those ideas, we turn toward a discussion of evidence-based practice. The research process, like the nursing process, is one of the tools we use to help us make decisions and solve problems. After a while, I expand the research discussion with a hypothetical case: "What happens if you purchase a shampoo and wash your hair and it turns green?"

This is a good time to reinforce the steps of both the nursing process and the research process. Hair turning green is an important piece of data. Even if the shampoo was recommended by an authority figure (a respected friend, perhaps), the data would lead the buyer to question its use. You can extend this situation to the authority figure in the clinical area (nurse educator or experienced nurse) who recommends a nursing intervention.

Nursing research can determine the effectiveness of an intervention without relying on customs and beliefs about nursing practice. Discussing the need for continued nursing research, tight research designs, and replication studies is an effective way to relate nursing research and nursing practice.

Ideas for Use

- Ask students to consider the influence of television, radio, and print media on different types of decision-making.
- You can ask students about any product they choose to purchase and use that item to describe the decision-making process. Personalize your teaching by using an object someone brought to class—a cell phone, laptop, or PDA, for example.
- Begin the discussion with the ways of knowing. Compare literature, customs, policies, peers, faculty, intuition, family members, or other experts with the research process as a way to validate knowledge.

- **How Do You Pick Your Shampoo?** is a playful way to open a research discussion with both students and practicing nurses.

Issues in Measurement

General Description   This strategy uses practical methods to teach measurement concepts, including reliability (consistency) and validity (accuracy). The exercises demonstrate the differences between these concepts and their relevance to the research process. See Froman and Owen[1] for examples in addition to those presented here and for details about each exercise.

Preparation and Equipment   In the measuring exercise each group of four students needs one 6- or 12-inch ruler, a 3-foot piece of string, a 1-foot piece of elastic, a pencil, and a tape measure. You may want to hand out "data sheets" to each student. See Table 7–1 for an example.

Example of the Strategy at Work   I've used **Issues in Measurement** with both staff development and nursing student classes. I split the class into groups of four. After I distributed the equipment and gave instructions,

Table 7–1. Head Measurement Data Sheet			
	Head A	**Head B**	**Head C**
Tape measure			
Ruler			
String			
Elastic			

each student measured the three other heads in the groups using the supplies I'd given out. No other directions were provided.

When all the measurements were completed, the group discussed the validity of each method used to obtain a head circumference. They related each method to the types of measurement used in the clinical area. The group also identified the difficulties of using a straight ruler to measure head circumference, the inaccuracies of measuring with elastic, and the interference caused by different hair styles and types of hair.

Ideas for Use

- This active, entertaining strategy gets students out of their chairs and involved in exercises.
- You can use both metric and standard measurement rulers and then discuss the discrepancies that result from using different units of measurement.

Reliability and Validity Darts

General Description   This is a general strategy that helps students differentiate reliability and validity. The reader is also referred to Froman and Owen[1] for additional details. **Reliability and Validity Darts** depicts the differences between validity (accuracy) and reliability (consistency).

Preparation and Equipment   Prepare a slide or sign that resembles Figure 7–1. Use it during class discussion to explain the concepts of reliability and validity.

Example of the Strategy at Work   You can let your slide work for you to illustrate how reliability and validity work. The darts are self-explanatory within the context of measurement issues.

Ideas for Use

- Include the diagram on a test. Students can indicate in pictures whether they understand the concepts of reliability and validity. Alternatively, they can discuss these concepts in an essay question or a short written assignment.
- Ask students to create their own diagrams depicting the concepts of reliability and validity.

Mock Studies

General Description   Students plan and carry out studies that reinforce concepts used in research. These include protection of human

RELIABILITY AND VALIDITY DARTS

**No Reliability
No Validity**

**Reliable,
Not Valid**

Reliable and Valid

Fig. 7–1.   Reliability and validity diagram.

subjects, data collection, analysis and interpretation, and nursing implications. The **Mock Study** and its conclusions illustrate the value of nursing research and evidence-based practice.

Preparation and Equipment   **Mock Studies** require a considerable amount of equipment. You'll need a blackboard, overhead projector, dry erase board, or flipchart to gather ideas.

Example of the Strategy at Work   One class I taught couldn't seem to appreciate the need for nursing research. We were talking about things that "bug" us in clinical practice. One student brought up her concerns about performing chest percussion on postoperative clients. She wondered whether the risks (pain inflicted) were outweighed by the benefits (mobilization of secretions) in these clients. Her question turned on a light bulb for me. Suddenly I saw how to create a study that would interest these students.

I let the class decide on the problem and the research question. Then I split them into groups of three or four and gave each group an assignment. These included designing the study, developing a sampling plan, discussing the literature review, anticipating issues with human subjects and data collection, considering methods of data analysis, understanding the conclusions, and tracking the dissemination of the results. The class quickly learned the interconnections of each step of the research process and understood the need for regular communication between groups.

Ideas for Use

- Ask your students to identify an area of conflict or questionable practice in the clinical area. Use this assignment as preparation for a future class.
- Have students do the assignment individually as an **Ah-hah Journal** or **E-mail Exercise.**
- Extend the assignment by asking students to identify a clinical issue, conduct a review of the literature, and propose research designs.

Group Research Critique

General Description   In this strategy, the instructor divides the class into pairs, trios, or small groups. These groups then select and critique a research article. They may use a specific format, found in nursing research texts, or simply discuss the positive and negative aspects of the article. This strategy is also valuable for highlighting current science during coverage of a clinical content topic.

Preparation and Equipment   A critiquing format is essential to this exercise. Most research texts include one. You can also find a format in Herrman, *The Critique Process for the Nursing Research Consumer,*[2] available from the Delaware Nurses Association. Make sure you use a format that meets the needs of the group and the level of detail needed for this assignment.

Although many different formats exist, most are fundamentally similar, asking the reader to appraise the study and evaluate its validity. Class content can also reinforce critiquing skills.

Example of the Strategy at Work   **Group Research Critique** works well if students are given a critiquing format. Sometimes I let students pick their own article, which increases their level of interest in the assignment, and sometimes I assign one. Having the entire class critique the same one or two articles ensures that you, the instructor, are well versed in the articles' assets and weaknesses. If students pick their own, I ask to approve it to make sure it is a nursing research article. If you do this, you may generate a discussion around the question, "What is nursing research?"

I've also used one article through the entire course or program. We refer to it as the class learns different research steps: design, data collection, analysis, interpretation, and so on. Students prepare for class by critiquing a certain element or the entire work; class discussion can then reinforce concepts. Even some basic concepts, such as "Is the study qualitative or quantitative?," may be unclear during this process. Class discussion provides an opportunity to clarify concepts and reinforce lecture material.

Ideas for Use

- **Group Research Critique** can help you teach the different aspects of a research article.
- You can use the article critique as the final examination.
- In hospital education, nurses can critique articles individually and then discuss them in group meetings or journal clubs.
- In agency education, **Group Research Critique** can enhance a class on research consumerism and application.
- Staff nurses can select articles appropriate to conditions they see often in their client population. Results of several articles or meta-analyses may be referred to agency practice or standard committees.
- Participants can discuss the value of research application. How might their personal nursing practice change as a result of their reading and critiquing nursing research? Their practice may not change immediately. However, it's valuable to examine the influence of research on the ways in which nurses practice and gain knowledge.

Clinical Application of Findings to Case Studies

General Description   The instructor asks students to find a nursing research article that applies to their personal nursing practice. A general case study leads them through evaluating the merit of the article.

Emphasis may be on the critique of the research and on the ability to use the results in clinical nursing practice.

Preparation and Equipment   Use the case study and questions that follow or develop your own. Ask the students to bring a nursing research article to the class or program.

Example of the Strategy at Work   I asked my students to bring an article of interest and to read it through once before class. In class I distributed the following case study and questions. The students were asked to consider the questions individually for 15 minutes; then we discussed them as a group.

Answering Questions Through Research

You are a practicing nurse with a strong foundation in evidence-based practice. You have a question about a nursing intervention common on your unit and decide to research the science behind that intervention. Use the information in your article to answer the following questions:

1. After one reading of the article, what nursing problem or practice do you think this study addresses?
2. After one reading of the article, what changes would you make in your personal nursing practice?
3. Now look more closely at your article. What information supports a change in practices, policies, or procedures?
4. Now review your article for weaknesses. Focus on the population, sample, sample size, methods, data collection, data-analysis techniques, or conclusions. How does this information have an impact on the potential changes you would make in your personal nursing practice?
5. What does this exercise teach you about critiquing nursing research and evidence-based practice?

Ideas for Use

- You may need to reinforce the importance of nursing research and its components. This lesson is important in itself.
- You can use **Clinical Application of Findings** after a critiquing exercise. This approach reinforces the need to appraise research before using its results to change nursing practice.

- Liven up the case study by adapting it for application to specific nursing specialties.
- Use a case study to illustrate the ethical issues that surround the research process and the role of the nurse as client advocate in research studies. You can present the following case to generate discussion about the ethical and legal aspects of research in regard to clients. Discussing these issues provides an interesting angle for both students and practicing nurses.

Deceiving the Client

Legal and Ethical Issues in Research

Immediately after a diagnosis of ovarian cancer, a client is offered chemotherapy with an experimental drug. In this research protocol, neither the effectiveness nor the side effects of the drug are known. The client was given a written description of the drug's action and effects before her nurse and physician asked her to sign the consent form. The client did not ask questions about the chemotherapy and felt obligated to accept this treatment because the physician offered no other choices. During 6 months of treatment, she weakened dramatically and at times seemed incoherent. The chemotherapy was continued despite the deterioration in the client's physical and mental condition.

Use this case to illustrate the nurse's role as client advocate and as proponent of research. It's a great way to generate a discussion on research, advances in medical science, and associated ethical dilemmas.

Research Moments in Every Class

General Description   This strategy reflects the principle that nursing research should be introduced into every area of content. For clinical and nonclinical information, the instructor briefly shares current research with the students. A focus on nursing implications highlights the need for evidence-based practice.

Preparation and Equipment   Before class, take a moment to quickly search an electronic full-text database. Use "research" as one of your key words to ensure that you access a study about a content area.

Example of the Strategy at Work   I've found **Research Moments** especially effective for relating research findings to current practice. An active

Box 7–3.
Research Moment

Examples of Current Research About Cystic Fibrosis
- Avoidance of summer camps for groups of children with CF (to prevent cross-infection).
- Screening of carriers and affected individuals to assist with early diagnosis and treatment. Implications for genetic counseling.
- Success of heart or lung transplants/quality of life for patients with CF.
- Genetic manipulation to enhance diagnosis and treatment.

search for each class topic reinforces the value of research and evidence-based practice.

I've used this method in many classes, including a class on cystic fibrosis (Box 7–3). A quick literature review yielded several articles related to current research. I summarized their content briefly on a slide, which led to a short discussion.

Ideas for Use

- In continuing education programs, **Research Moments** helps to relate findings to current, local practices.
- You can encourage attentiveness in your students by telling them they'll be tested on research results. Then include a question about the research in a comprehensive examination.
- Ask your students to research topics related to daily class content. If the class is small enough, they can share their results with the group. When their peers become research information finders, other students will discover incentive to apply research to their own practice.

Research Corners—Electronic or Bulletin Board

General Description   **Research Corners** resembles the **Research Moments** strategy. The difference is that abstracts and interesting findings are posted either on cork boards or electronically. Like **Research Moments,** this strategy doesn't take much time.

Preparation and Equipment   You'll need a bulletin board if you plan to post research results on paper. For electronic postings, use a Web-based platform that allows attachments to a page that the class can view.

Example of the Strategy at Work   **Research Corners** enhances knowledge of a content area while reinforcing the need for nursing research. For physical postings, I either type a brief summary of an article or cut the abstract out of a journal. Interesting clip art and colors add to the visual appeal of the board. Citations are kept brief and are limited to interesting findings at the students' level. For electronic postings, I attach summaries or abstracts to the class page for viewing.

Ideas for Use

- Allow students to provide research ideas, abstracts, or summaries for posting.
- Use **Research Corners** as either a required or an extra credit assignment.
- Use bulletin boards to promote research in break rooms or common nursing areas.
- Use **Online Discussion Groups** to discuss current research findings.
- Provide incentives to encourage staff or students to develop visual displays about a particular topic. Encourage them to change these displays frequently. Students can receive extra credit for assignments. Staff nurses can be given clinical ladder credit, agency "freebies," or books to reward their participation.
- Brief, eye-catching messages are important for busy nurses and students.
- A colleague posts **Research Corners** on her door, making a statement about nursing research and providing reading material for visitors.

Film Clips in Nursing Research

General Description   The instructor shows clips of current films to stimulate discussion of research concepts. These film clips should delineate a problem or issue in current research or health care.

Preparation and Equipment   You'll need a supply of video or DVD clips, cued to specific scenes. Before class, you'll need to establish objectives for the exercise, consider the questions you'll ask, and speculate on areas for future investigation.

Example of the Strategy at Work   Many popular films raise issues that nursing research can and should address. (for guidelines, see the **Short Clips** section of Chapter 3). After showing a short clip, I ask the class to formulate a research question or develop a research design addressing the topic. I've used clips to illustrate the steps of the research process, to stimulate research ideas, and to make research "real" from a movie perspective.

Ideas for Use

- Potential film topics include specific illnesses, clients dealing with symptoms, legal and ethical dilemmas, and social science content.
- Ask the class how nursing research might have changed the outcome of the film clip.
- Have students develop a **Mock Study** based on the research questions derived from a film clip.
- After showing a clip, use **E-mail Exercises** or **Ah-hah Journals** to brainstorm ideas for research design.

Clinical Area Questioning—Research at Work

General Description   Clinical instructors are attuned to the value of research. In this strategy, the instructor investigates the literature to determine what is known about a topic and then presents the findings to the class. Clinical and practice issues present an opportunity for **Clinical Area Questioning.**

Preparation and Equipment   To begin with, you need an inquiring mind in the clinical area. The clinical question or issue determines the need to research the literature and find out what is known about the topic.

Example of the Strategy at Work   Students and staff nurses were asking questions about a clinical problem. A client had been admitted with a diagnosis of aspiration pneumonia. This client had been receiving nasogastric tube feedings at home.

I saw this situation as a great opportunity to demonstrate the value of nursing research. A literature review discovered studies that addressed ways of checking nasogastric tube placement. Auscultation of air injected into a tube, aspiration of gastric contents, pH of gastric contents, and chest x-ray were compared for feasibility, effectiveness, and other criteria. Our summary of the findings generated much discussion about local practice and the procedures recommended by nursing textbooks.

Ideas for Use

- Ask unit instructors, senior clinical ladder nurses, or student leaders to do literature searches and disseminate information.
- Information may be posted on electronic bulletin boards or cork boards.
- Like **Research Moments in Every Class, Clinical Area Questioning** should be inherent in every clinical experience.
- Keep a log of questions asked in day-to-day clinical practice so you can research problems later on.

- Ask students to determine their own clinical problems or issues to be researched and examined.
- Colleagues used this strategy to share "Nursing Research Myth Busters" with fellow nurses. Clinical questions from the group list serv were used to stimulate research, gather evidence, and come to practice-based conclusions. By using the questions and issues from active bedside practice, participants not only received information valuable to enhancing patient care but also saw the value of investigation to solve clinical problems and the potential for research to improve patient outcomes.

Paper Towel Ideas

General Description   In this strategy, a common roll of paper towels can inspire creative thinking. Students list their ideas, one per sheet, unrolling the towels as their ideas evolve.

Preparation and Equipment   You'll need one roll of paper towels for each individual, pair, trio, or group. Each roll needs a marker for writing down ideas. For added incentive, you can bring in prizes to reward the greatest number of ideas. **Paper Towel Ideas** is a relatively inexpensive strategy.

Example of the Strategy at Work   A colleague asks students to use up their paper towels by listing researchable ideas, one to a sheet. Other faculty have used this strategy in research groups to list other concepts, such as types of sampling criteria and methods of data collection.

Ideas for Use

- You can give prizes to the individuals or groups who come up with the greatest number of ideas, measured in the number of paper towels they unroll.
- The competitive atmosphere stimulates different, creative ideas.
- You can use **Paper Towel Ideas** any time you want to brainstorm ideas and come up with new thoughts.
- Some faculty use toilet paper to create lists. Others reject this variation on the strategy, attaching a negative connotation to the use of toilet paper.
- You can use **Paper Towel Ideas** at the beginning and end of a course or program to demonstrate how far the students' thinking has evolved.

Faculty Research Sharing

General Description   Instructors share personal nursing research experience to demonstrate that professionals participate in and are invested in research. Unlike **War Stories and Clinical Anecdotes,** this strategy focuses on research concepts rather than day-to-day clinical experience. **Faculty Research Sharing** works well in any class.

Preparation and Equipment   You may want to use slides or overheads to describe research findings.

Example of the Strategy at Work   **Faculty Research Sharing** illustrates important concepts and highlights the challenges and rewards of research. In my experience, it's better for students to hear brief discussions without elaborate discourses on design and implementation. For example, when differentiating quantitative and qualitative data, I avoided a theoretical discussion and stuck to examples from personal research.

Ideas for Use

- Maintain a focus on research concepts and keep **Faculty Research Sharing** brief and relevant to class content.
- As you share your research, make sure to keep the presentation at the knowledge level of the students.
- Have other speakers or faculty share their research experiences with the class.
- You can take as little as 10 minutes to share research findings. Presented in the middle of a class, they can reinforce the importance of research in any clinical area.
- Clinical experts can share a policy or practice that was developed or changed on the basis of clinical research.
- When discussing in-depth data analysis procedures or complex theoretical frameworks, take care not to "turn off" the students.
- Ask faculty or guest speakers to discuss a single step of the research process—consent of human subjects, data collection, and so on—to keep the focus on class objectives.

Poster Sessions

General Description   Student groups create a poster based on a research article or a review of several articles. The research must reflect a practice issue. Because the posters are based on specific criteria and resemble those displayed at professional meetings, they prepare both students and nurses for scholarly presentation.

Preparation and Equipment   You should develop a specific grading rubric or evaluation criterion for submissions. The students contribute poster boards, illustrations, information, and the effort of making the poster.

Example of the Strategy at Work   Colleagues have used **Poster Sessions** in research and continuing education classes to promote active participation and research evaluation. One colleague split a class into groups of five. Each group picked its own topic and found an article or review. Students used the assignment criteria to critique the study and used the posters to display their analysis. Afterward the instructor graded the posters.

Some of my colleagues have organized a poster display day. Student posters are graded, and the best ones win a small prize or award. Students also work individually with faculty on literature reviews, **Mock Studies,** or pilot studies and present their results in a **Poster Session.**

Ideas for Use

- Invite your colleagues to the poster displays. They can help you evaluate posters and assist in disseminating the students' research findings.
- In the clinical area, assign units to complete a quality-improvement activity, a literature review, or a pilot study. Then have them develop posters. Display the posters during nurses' week or in conjunction with an educational program. Provide rewards and recognition for participants.
- Encourage students and nurses attending conferences to view and evaluate research posters created by other nurses.
- Encourage students to submit posters to local conferences that foster student involvement in research.

Research Concept Maps

General Description   Visual maps of research concepts and methods are used to reinforce the research process or to critique individual studies. See Rooda[3] for the use of mind mapping in a research course.

Preparation and Equipment   For individual assignments, you'll need drawing supplies or software that can generate concept maps. For class or group concept mapping, you can use a blackboard, dry-erase board, overhead projector, or flipchart. If an entire class or large group is working on one poster, spread a large sheet of paper over a desk or table so they can all contribute to the concept map.

Example of the Strategy at Work   I've had students map out the research process on the blackboard. As with any concept map exercise, lines can be drawn to show connections between concepts reflected in circles or squares. Colors, shapes, and placement on the map can represent categories, steps, or differences in concepts. Concepts may be as elaborate or as simple as desired. See Rooda[3] for examples of research concept maps.

Ideas for Use

- You can use **Research Concept Maps** with pairs, trios, or groups.
- Try using the strategy as a test question: ask students to draw the research process.
- Design a homework project in which students critique an article using a concept map.

Campus or Unit Research and Nurse Interviews

General Description   Students survey peers and other students to learn the elements of tool development, field research, observational research, and data analysis. Practicing nurses can live the experience of data collection by polling each other on selected information. During their clinical rotations, students interview staff nurses about the use of nursing research in the clinical area. Practicing nurses ask colleagues similar questions. These interviews can be either formal or informal.

Preparation and Equipment   No equipment is needed. Students or nurses may conduct interviews before a scheduled class discussion. Interviewers should agree on topics to make sure that all interviews are on similar subjects. You may want to consider topics ahead of time to help your students brainstorm ideas for interviews.

Example of the Strategy at Work   I've used this strategy early in a course or program to determine the research climate in which nurses work and the local attitudes toward evidence-based practice. Students can generate questions and then discuss their interviews in subsequent sessions.

An effective single question is, "Do you use research to guide your nursing practice?" I've also expanded this question to include such areas as level of research education, participation in policy and procedure development, reading of nursing journals, and involvement in research studies. I've asked students and nurses to conduct informal studies of their peers. For student peer interviews, I sometimes pick a topic before class and instruct the students to "ask around" about that topic. They can use sample questions or develop their own.

For nursing students, topics should reflect daily life. I've instructed students to ask as many people as possible if they shower in the morning, in the evening, or at some other time. Early in the spring semester, I've asked students to poll peers about their plans for spring break. For practicing nurses, demographic surveys may be valuable.

My students conduct interviews either alone or in pairs. We tabulate the results in a subsequent class. This method allows us to explore the data collection and analysis phases of research.

Ideas for Use

- **Campus or Unit Research** can be combined with **Mock Studies** to simulate study design and implementation.
- This strategy can generate enthusiastic interest in nursing research at the unit or group level.
- On a unit, you may want to include nurse managers, physicians, and clinical specialists in the interviews.
- According to the local research climate, this method may highlight the need for increased evidence-based practice in clinical settings.
- Nurses may claim that they don't use research in daily practice. You can guide a student's line of questioning with such queries as "How does your agency come up with policies and procedures?," "How does your unit conduct quality assurance?," and "How do standards of care change a client's course of stay in the hospital?" These questions may uncover a deeper appreciation of evidence-based practice for both the student interviewer and the practicing nurse.
- **Campus or Unit Research** makes a good icebreaker. Ask students to poll their peers on a topic and then use their findings to stimulate a discussion.
- You can use this strategy to explain different types of data and the methods used to organize them.
- Descriptive statistics, such as mean, mode, and median, can be calculated and discussed as data descriptors.

In the Know

General Description   The tabloids in the grocery store have taught us that human nature reacts to the different, exceptional, and outrageous. Although not all nursing research findings meet these criteria, research sometimes uncovers surprising results that warrant further study and exploration. These are the facts that will catch your students' attention in class. **In the Know** requires the instructor to be in tune with these data and to be able to summarize them simply.

Presenting a potential medical or nursing advance, much like those announced on the evening news, provides an opportunity for discussion and a point of interest. Of course, validity and reliability should be weighed before the data are accepted as fact. This critical process is educational in itself.

Preparation and Equipment   Follow the introduction of research information to the lay public, peruse research journals, or do your own quick study of current research. Any of these methods can provide insights that will engage your students' thinking. You must include the source and validity of that information to avoid misconceptions or misunderstandings.

Example of the Strategy at Work   The newspaper frequently publishes information about current scientific research. Issues such as stem cell research, medical advances, and development of new medications are part of everyday news. Interestingly, busy nurses and nursing students are sometimes so absorbed with work and study that they are insulated from the news.

Current events that affect nursing practice or exemplify nursing research are especially useful. Recent exposés of widespread errors in medication administration have created a public outcry and call for a change in health-care practices. Clearly, changes are needed to ensure cautious and careful medication administration and eliminate inferior standards of care. Being **In the Know** about such findings is an important way to validate good practice. Discussing these studies and their nursing implications underlines to students the importance of prudent nursing practice.

Ideas for Use

- **In the Know** may be used to discuss both sound and unsound research. Encourage your students to analyze any method or interpretation they find questionable.
- This strategy is a great way to reinforce the fascinating nature of research and scientific inquiry.
- Use **In the Know** to discuss the need for replication of nursing studies. In addition, replication with varying samples is necessary to ensure that results can be generalized. It's important to emphasize that changes in practice should occur only after findings are validated and the literature has been reviewed thoroughly.
- Students can search public media to find **In the Know** topics. These topics can be collected as an **Admit Ticket,** written about in a short assignment, or used to guide class discussion.

- Assign groups to review the media portrayal of current advances in disease treatment. Thanks to the Internet, we can view archival news clips to learn what the lay public has been told about a medical issue. These clips are often generated from large-scale studies in reputable nursing and medical journals. Students can compare the public information with the scientific study to determine the accuracy of the portrayal, the implications for nursing practice, and the need for further study.

Bring on the Evidence

General Description   Nurses and nursing students at every level are hearing about the importance of evidence-based practice. Novices often have trouble understanding what data count as evidence and how to assess their validity. Sometimes information is accepted as truth because the messenger has a convincing manner, not because the information has been appraised accurately. **Bring on the Evidence** allows students to function as "research sleuths" on a clinical or nursing issue.

Students select or are assigned a clinical problem or research dilemma. They develop the research question, essentially conducting a literature review. The difference is that the students are uncovering and collecting research evidence in a "private detective" style.

Preparation and Equipment   You may want to use **Bring on the Evidence** as a final project for a research class. You need to develop the assignment, determine how many grade points you'll award for different aspects of the work, and develop a list of potential clinical issues or problems.

Example of the Strategy at Work   This strategy is especially valuable for smaller classes or clinical groups. The assignment may be done alone or as a group activity; I've found that groups work especially well.

First, students select a clinical problem or issue. During the first class session we discuss and define this topic, and the class brainstorms potential key words to use in a search. The brainstorming session and choice of key words are essential, especially for novice researchers. I like to organize a field trip to the library, or at least to a computer that allows access to library databases. This type of practice provides a certain level of comfort with the research process.

I encourage my students to print full-text articles and to access articles "the old way"—by going to the library stacks and finding the article in a bound journal. Students can list their evidence and bring the list to class. Subsequent classes review the evidence and discuss implications for further research and nursing practice.

Ideas for Use

- Students can present their evidence as a **Poster Session** accompanied by a short discussion of their conclusions.
- In a clinical setting, students can use the policies and procedures of the unit to generate their clinical issue. They can then **Bring on the Evidence** to inform the unit staff about their findings and to recommend further inquiry to the agency procedure committees.
- Students may frame their evidence as an **In-class Debate,** presenting their research findings versus a traditional or institutional practice. Ask them to analyze the evidence and to decide whether it's time to recommend a change in practice.
- Award prizes to students who find the most definitive evidence.
- This strategy may be combined with a **Mock Trial** to continue the "sleuth" theme.

Author Guidelines

General Description   Once students appreciate the value of nursing research, they discover an incentive to become research consumers themselves. The **Author Guidelines** strategy simulates the experience of developing a manuscript for publication. This strategy is meant to be coupled with other projects to teach the next step in the research process—dissemination.

Students use an original research idea or some other project to explore the publication process. The project can be a **Campus or Unit Research Interview, Mock Study,** or any other strategy that replicates the research process.

Author Guidelines takes that strategy a step further. Students review current journals that would potentially publish their idea and bring the author guidelines for that journal to class. Alternatively, the instructor can download or obtain author guidelines to be distributed in class.

Preparation and Equipment   Preparation begins with another assignment related to the research process. You can use one of the other research strategies described in this chapter.

Example of the Strategy at Work   **Campus or Unit Research** and **Mock Studies** are the best foundation for preparing a simulated manuscript. After designing and completing the first step of the process, students then use their **Author Guidelines** to complete a short assignment. They can write the abstract, lay out the sections of the article, or develop an outline of the potential manuscript. Encourage your students to review the guidelines for specific requirements, such as formatting, length, and audience. Many editors suggest reviewing other articles in the journal to learn its literary style.

I've used **Author Guidelines** to discuss the difference between writing school papers and writing for journals (a challenge for many of us). I also emphasize the importance of meeting the needs of the audience. This is a good time to discuss the peer-review process, acceptance rates, the challenges of writing for publication, and opportunities to begin a career in writing. Letters to the editor, any type of commentary, smaller community and local nursing publications, and professional organizations all provide good opportunities for the beginning writer.

Ideas for Use

- This assignment can be adapted for a group activity, a single homework assignment, or a class writing exercise.
- Students can compare the author guidelines of different journals to discover the particular priorities of each publication.
- Classes can peruse issues of a journal to get a feeling for its target audience. Encourage discussion questions such as "Who is this journal designed for?," "How does the audience determine the writing style?," and "How much research is published in this journal?" Discussion questions can be reviewed in pairs and trios to encourage participation.
- Advanced students can use **Author Guidelines** to develop concept papers for publication or assist faculty with research, leading to a joint publication.
- Have your students draft a query letter for a particular journal using the **Author Guidelines** or journal rules.

References

1. Froman RD, and Owen, SV: Teaching reliability and validity: Fun with classroom application. Journal of Continuing Education in Nursing 22:88–94, 1991.
2. Herrman, J: The Critique Process for the Nursing Research Consumer. Delaware Nurses Association, Newark, DE, 1999.
3. Rooda, LA: Effects of mind mapping on student achievement in a nursing research course. Nurse Educator 19:25–27, 1994.

Personal Journal Pages

Chapter 8
Conclusion

"Teaching was the hardest work I have ever done, and it remains the hardest work I have done to date." —Ann Richards

"My joy in learning is partly that it enables me to teach" —Seneca

"Every one of us is both a student and a teacher." —S. Johnson and C. Johnson

General Hints for Using Creative Strategies

Start Out Slowly

This book is full of ideas that you can creatively add to your personal teaching style and the content of your class. Always use creative strategies in moderation. The class that's barraged with too many strategies and innovative methods will experience "creativity fatigue." One to three strategies per class or session is probably enough to introduce the concept of collaborative learning.

Small doses of creative strategy will also keep you from forcing uncomfortable learning styles on your students. This caution is especially important for students accustomed to passive learning styles and noninteractive teaching. Your students may need time to get comfortable with their own involvement and their need to participate actively in the teaching-learning process. If a class is reluctant to transform its own learning practices, you can choose some of the more personal and less collaborative teaching strategies, such as those that involve personal introspection and writing. By beginning with less threatening strategies, you may eventually progress to more active ones. Remember to use any kind of strategy sparingly to keep methods innovative and fun.

Active learning methods can be difficult to introduce into a nursing curriculum. Students used to academic settings may prefer a passive, spoonfeeding approach to learning. "Just tell me what's on the test" is the motto for some of these students. Professional nursing groups may be fatigued and regard class time as a reprieve from the demands of client care. They may prefer just listening to participating in a creative strategy. Again, choose your strategies judiciously and add them sparingly.

More Ideas for Groups

Nurse learners may or may not be responsive to working in groups. One of the biggest hurdles in such work is to assign the groups initially. If your class time is limited, you may choose to establish the groups in advance. This approach gives you a chance to split up cliques and ensure the same skill and experience level in each group. Also, students who don't know each other are spared the embarrassment of grouping themselves. You can often facilitate small group work simply by using seat placement in the room. See **Group Thought** for more hints on group work.

Set the Rules

Not only do creative teaching strategies stimulate learning, but they also engender activity, excitement, and discussion. At the outset you need to establish ground rules that specify how to carry out each strategy, the time frame for each activity, and your expectations for student participation and behavior. You'll need signals to initiate creative strategies and to indicate a return to more traditional methods, which call for quiet listening. Some instructors use a whistle or some other sound to signal transitions. You must also allow time for transitions between strategies. Some spontaneous conversation and activity during the transitions is to be expected.

Not all strategies will be well received or embraced by every student. Learning style, generation, cultural norms, and personality traits all influence a student's response to teaching strategies. Encourage total participation, but respect your students by trying to make your teaching comfortable for all of them.

Develop Your Style

Make sure you are knowledgeable and well versed in the content before you integrate creative teaching strategies. The first time you present on a topic may not be the time to implement elaborate strategies. Instead, engage students by using one or two simple collaborative strategies. Focus on delivering organized content that your students can understand. Subsequent teaching will provide more opportunities to use creative methods.

Most important, as you add strategies to your teaching portfolio, you'll develop a teaching style unique to your personality. You must be comfortable with your methods to convey an active learning message to the class. Use the strategies in this book as a springboard to creating new and different teaching methods. Not only should students be having fun with creative strategies, you should too. If teaching becomes laborious, it's time to re-energize yourself by assessing your methods and possibly revising your strategies.

Make Learning Fun

Humor needs to be funny—obviously. As a teacher, you carry the burden of making sure that everybody can laugh at your humor. It must be politically correct, without offensive words or connotations, culturally appropriate, and generally understandable to the class. If you aren't sure whether something is offensive, don't use it. Chances are that you'll offend someone if you do.

Humor changes the pace in a teaching session, reinforces ideas, promotes retention, and puts content on a human plane. When class content is fun to learn and to teach, your students get the idea that you like to teach and are excited to be doing so. Paulson[1] offers a great guide to humor in the workplace (see also the Annotated Bibliography).

Advantages and Disadvantages of Creative Strategies

The major advantage of creative teaching strategies is the ability to reel in the students and get them to enjoy learning. An instructor can best reach a student by combining creativity, teaching skills, and knowledge of the content. Creative strategies facilitate transitions from one topic to another and appeal to diverse learning styles. They help students connect their knowledge with their experience, encourage lasting retention of material, and stimulate discussion and reflection.

Creative strategies have their disadvantages. You take a risk with each method: it may work well or it may "crash and burn." Planning and preparation time may be significant. Also, creative strategies can drain the class time needed to cover content.

Some students may prefer more passive learning methods. Others may not connect the purpose of the exercise with the class content. They may misconstrue information, not appreciate its significance, or neglect to apply lessons from the exercise to their theoretical knowledge and nursing practice. Some students may regard creative strategies as unprofessional or childish, unrelated to the knowledge they need to function as professional nurses. Finally, your greatest challenge may be the time and effort required to change your teaching habits and launch your students outside their comfort zone.

That being said, you as instructor have the choice of using as many creative strategies as you feel comfortable with. You're not trying to overhaul your entire way of teaching, just to spice it up a little. That's the beauty of this book. It's up to you whether to employ one or 100 strategies in your years as a teacher.

Finding the Teaching Fuel

You will be able to find "teaching fuel" in some of the most unexpected places. Quotations and stories may come from magazines, books, calendars, e-mail, quotation anthologies, or colleagues. Ideas will come to you in the shower, at a stop light, or when you're falling asleep at night. Anything thought provoking, funny, or relevant, or any **Ah-hah,** is potential class material.

When looking for teaching fuel, keep your professionalism in mind. Remember the key rules of borrowing from others: adhere to fair use laws and cite known sources to give credit where it's due. Seek strategies in unlikely places and share them with others.

Guidelines for PowerPoint

PowerPoint has changed the way we teach, especially in the lecture format. It lets teachers connect with the Internet during a lecture, linking to Web sites and other online resources. We all know a picture is worth a thousand words. Scanning in photographs, drawings, other graphics, and charts from articles or textbooks helps us appeal to the visual learner. We can also incorporate movie clips, clip art, and animation. Downloading songs and subject-specific sounds, such as heart and breath sounds, provides a valuable experience for the whole class and especially for auditory learners.

Using PowerPoint, we can download handouts from a remote source or through Web-based educational platforms. Handout formats vary, so you can choose the ones you prefer. Blank formats save printer ink and download time. The use of computer and LCD technology provides audiovisual materials that many students can access simultaneously. This method, which is usually reliable, frees students from the burden of taking copious notes. Slide-based notes appeal especially to auditory learners, who can focus on listening rather than write furiously without taking in the material.

A PowerPoint presentation helps you steer the course of your class, keep the lecture on track, and maintain the pace. It can guide both you and your students by highlighting key areas within the class content. In contrast, PowerPoint must be used judiciously and with some caution. The class or lecture is only as good as the instructor. No amount of fancy graphics will compensate for a teacher who doesn't know the subject well. PowerPoint is an instructional tool, not a crutch to get teachers through unfamiliar material. Here are some hints to make PowerPoint an even more effective tool in your teaching portfolio:

- Make sure you use at least a 24-point font on your slides.
- Use a single font throughout a presentation. For emphasis, use upper- and lower-case letters, bold type, underlining, shading, and italics.
- Use the custom animation function to focus on key words. Animation can be used at the beginning or end of a presentation or to emphasize a word at any point. You can change settings to vary any available effects, including animation and the prompt to start it. Be careful not to overuse this function.
- Slide transition animation, used when you advance to the next slide, offers interesting formats. Use the random transition setting for a different type of transition with each slide.
- Use dark backgrounds with light lettering for larger classes. Experiment with different slide designs and color schemes to find what works best with specific class content.

- Don't use too many slides. As a general rule, you should lecture at least 1 to 2 minutes for every slide. For complex or technical topics, one slide every 4 to 5 minutes may be the maximum number to use in your lecture.

- When writing a class lecture, use caution if you're making the slides concurrently. The temptation is to write all the lecture content on the slide. Instead, use the Note Page function for your lecture; the actual slides include only integral information.

- Slides should include prompts and bulleted ideas, not every fact discussed in class. The general rule is to limit a slide to six bullet points, with no more than six words per bullet. Include graphics and animation to increase interest (see earlier). Keep students actively engaged by leaving blanks in the slides for them to fill in during the presentation.

- For some students, PowerPoint handouts have replaced in-class note taking. Encourage your students to take notes related to class discussions, their questions, or interesting points used to augment the slides. For students who have trouble knowing what to write, suggest that they take class notes in their usual way. Then have them incorporate the PowerPoint notes into their written notes after class. This revisiting of material is especially helpful for visual and kinesthetic learners.

- Control the pace of your class. Allow for questions and pauses by not using automatic timing for slide transitions.

- Don't forget that a well-informed, experienced, and engaging teacher is worth far more than an elaborate slide presentation. The value of teacher-student interchange, discussion, and class attendance cannot be overemphasized.

Evaluate Your Strategies

We need a research foundation to support evidence-based nursing education. In the early years of nursing research, interest focused on how nurses learned and how to enhance learning. As research priorities became more focused on the client outcomes, funding for and emphasis on nursing education research diminished. Now the earlier interest has been renewed. The emphasis is on developing a better understanding of what works in nursing education, and on carrying evidence-based nursing focus from the practice setting into the nursing educational arena.

Readers are charged with conducting evaluative research as they use the creative strategies found in this book. Much of the evidence so far is anecdotal, based on instructor and student satisfaction with a teaching method.

The strategies in this book have all succeeded and appear intuitively to have a positive impact on learning. Few have undergone rigorous research to determine their true value.

As is noted by McCartney and Morin,[2] "Faculty need to find the best evidence for decision-making in education and no longer base their practice on time-honored tradition ("because we have always done it that way")." Several books listed in the Annotated Bibliography discuss the research available for selected innovative strategies. Most educational research includes small studies of students' responses to classroom innovations, pre- and post-intervention knowledge assessments, and retrospective measures associated with nursing program completion and NCLEX® success.

The publication of a new journal, *The International Journal of Nursing Education Scholarship*,[3] testifies to the present emphasis on nursing education research. To validate the infusion of new strategies into traditional methods, we need designs that go beyond personal satisfaction or individual perceptions of learning. Solid research designs, including quasi-experimental studies with equivalent control and treatment groups, may best determine the effectiveness of creative teaching methods.

I also ask you to share your experience of what worked and what didn't. This information is key to our evaluating the methods in this book and their use by nurse educators. The companion Web site for this book is the optimal forum for sharing and continued exploration of creative teaching strategies. The link is http://davisplus.fadavis.com/herrman. Your contributions to this Web site, from student responses to major research initiatives, will continue to build the foundation for evidence-based nursing education. Use this Web site to continue enhancing your teaching skills and, ultimately, your students' learning experience.

Some Words About Motivation

An appropriate way to close this book is with a common saying and a not-so-common addition to that phrase. In this book, I've tried to capture the art of innovative teaching. All of these creative strategies are intended to motivate learners and learning.

The old adage contends, "You can lead a horse to water, but you can't make it drink." This phrase has been expanded: "but you can feed it salty oats to make it thirsty (Fig. 8–1)." I hope the creative teaching strategies in this book will stimulate your students' thirst for knowledge and skills. I wish you well as you continue to teach, and to enhance learning in, today's and tomorrow's nursing professionals.

Fig. 8–1.   "You can lead a horse to water, but you can't make it drink."

References

1. Paulson, TL: Making Humor Work: Take Your Job Seriously and Yourself Lightly. Crisp Learning, Menlo Park, CA, 1989.
2. McCartney, PR, and Morin, KH: Where is the evidence for teaching methods used in nursing education. MCN The American Journal of Maternal Child Nursing 30(6):406–412, 2005.
3. The International Journal of Nursing Education. Scholarship Berkeley Electronic Press. Published monthly since 2004.

Personal Journal Pages

Annotated Bibliography

1. Bean, JC: Engaging Ideas: The Professor's Guide to Integrating Writing, Critical Thinking, and Active Learning in the Classroom. John Wiley & Sons, San Francisco, 2001.

   Description: This interesting book is designed to enhance classroom teaching. It focuses on the integration of writing, critical thinking, and active learning techniques into classroom activities.

   Features: A useful feature is the "executive summary" in the first chapter; it sums up the intent of the book. Chapters focus on connecting thought and writing; designing problem-based assignments; coaching students as learners, thinkers, and writers; and reading, commenting on, and grading student writing. Although innovative strategies are found throughout the book, most of them appear in the section on coaching. Thinking tasks and active classroom learning are described and examples are provided.

Innovative Strategies:

- *Ten Strategies for Designing Critical Thinking Tasks.* This section lists selected strategies and some components needed to design thinking exercises.
- *Believing and Doubting Strategy.* This strategy resembles **In-class Debate** except that each participant takes both sides of the controversy.
- *Guided Journal Tasks.* Concepts from lectures become subjects for journals and free writing in class.
- *Time Outs.* As in **Let's Discuss,** time is spent in discussing class content.
- *Paper Chase Questioning.* Students are questioned to encourage them to "think on their feet." This strategy is modeled on the movie *The Paper Chase,* although instructors are encouraged to use far more nurturing methods.
- *Out of Class Peer Review.* Students take home each other's paper drafts and bring them back to class with their feedback and evaluation.

2. Billings, DM, and Hallstead, JA: Teaching in Nursing: A Guide for Faculty, ed 2. Saunders, Philadelphia, 2005.

    Description: This book includes field-tested strategies for a variety of teaching settings. It provides a theoretical foundation for many of the strategies, as well as for techniques to enhance teaching and learning.

    Features: The chapters are divided into sections, such as Faculty and Students; Curriculum; Teaching and Learning; Teaching, Learning, and Information Resources; and Evaluation. Creative teaching strategies are woven throughout. Most of them appear in chapters on the enhancement of critical thinking, clinical teaching, and classroom assessment. The book can be used as both a nursing education text and a comprehensive resource for current nurse educators. Also provided is the *EVOLE* Web link to supplement the contents of the text.

Innovative Strategies:

- *The Learning Resource Center.* This hub of activity for student psychomotor learning includes audiovisuals, client simulators and mannequins, hospital supplies, computer resources, and teaching support specific to the learning resource center.
- *Computer Testing.* Students can use this valid, reliable, secure, and feasible testing method through the Web or other online resources.
- *Simulation Games.* Games are used to simulate an intense experience, such as aging, disability, injury, or a conflict.
- *Algorithms.* As in **Using Mnemonics,** teachers break complex procedures into steps and use strategies to encourage memorization.
- *Role Play.* Participants assume roles and act out scenarios to appreciate challenges and practice responses to selected issues.
- *Reflective Practice and Journaling.* Journals are used to assess learning; the authors reinforce the need for frequent instructor feedback.

3. Bradshaw, MJ, and Lowenstein, A: Innovative Teaching Strategies in Nursing and Related Health Professions, ed 4. Jones and Bartlett, Sudbury, MA, 2007.

    Description: This is the fourth edition of a classic resource for nurse educators. The latest edition builds on the previous ones, discussing when a lecture is not a lecture, simulations, creativity and humor, technology-assisted strategies, remote faculty, teaching of sensitive subjects, reflective practice, clinical teaching, futuristic techniques, and homemade strategies.

Features: Each chapter is filled with information about teaching in nursing. Creative strategies are scattered throughout the text, but most are in the chapters that relate to supplementing the lecture method.

Innovative Strategies:

- *The Delphi Technique.* This research method helps experts determine opinions and then reach consensus about an issue.
- *The Tree of Impact.* This strategy analyzes the possible consequences of a decision or an event.
- *Student-Selected Clinical Experiences.* This method helps students meet learning requirements and fulfill their specialty requests.
- *Portable Patient Problem Pack.* In this teaching-learning method, a card format is used to solve problems related to the nursing process.
- *Creativity in Nursing.* Suggestions are given for infusing poetry, literature, and other methods into nursing education.
- *High-Fidelity Patient Simulators.* This section discusses the current computerized patient simulators and describes signs and symptoms that may be replicated and changed with the available equipment.
- *Movement as Embodied Knowledge.* Movement and kinesiology can teach such concepts as self-awareness, family-client experiences, and reflective exploration.
- *Nursing Process Mapping Replaces Nursing Care Plans.* Traditional care plans are combined with concept maps.

4. Crisp Publications Series

Description: These books are part of the *50 Minute Series*, a set of more than 300 self-paced learning and personal exercise books. It offers a variety of titles related to teaching, management, computer skills, communication, leadership, public speaking, organizational skills, stress, time management, change, and personal growth.

Features: The books are designed to be "read with a pencil," making them suitable for different learning styles. Many books are also available on CD-ROM. The complete list of the books is available at www.thompson.com and www.courseilt.com. These sites also provide ordering information.

Innovative strategies: Each book has clear objectives, readings, exercises, quotations, and amusing cartoons to help make learning fun. Many of the exercises fit the "on the run" nature of nursing education. Following are the ones I have used. Some have been noted previously in this book

Lloyd, SR: Developing Positive Assertiveness. Crisp, Menlo Park, CA, 2001.

Maddux, RB: Team Building. Crisp, Menlo, Park, CA, 2004.

Mandel, S: Effective Presentation Skills. Crisp, Menlo, Park, CA, 2006.

Paulson, TL: Making Humor Work. Crisp, Menlo Park, CA, 1989.

5. Deck, ML: Instant Teaching Tools for the New Millennium. Mosby, St. Louis, 2004.

Deck, ML: More Instant Teaching Tools for Health Care Educators. Mosby, St. Louis, 1998.

Deck, ML: Instant Teaching Tools for Health Care Educators. Mosby, St. Louis, 1995.

Description: This unique series of books offers many creative strategies for nursing and health-care educators to add to their usual teaching methods. Games, crossword puzzles, and other activities make learning fun.

Features: Each teaching strategy is ready to use and easy to understand. Strategies may be revised to meet individual teaching needs. Each strategy includes the exercise, the time needed to complete it, the "tool box" or supplies needed, and helpful hints called "educator secrets." Guidelines help the teacher prepare and carry out each exercise. Prototypes for copying, quizzes, answer keys, and key terms are included for many of the exercises. These strategies may be used in academic education and staff development, and include interesting ways to teach mandatory skills and content in your institution. The books include many important hints, such as guides to using the templates and directions to help fit the strategy into busy working environments.

Innovative Strategies:

Examples of interesting exercises include:

- *Code Cart Contents Contest.* This strategy teaches nurses and other health-care personnel the location of code cart supplies, ensuring that staff can access them quickly.
- *People Bingo.* In this icebreaker, participants get to know each other by using premade bingo boards to find group members with matching selected characteristics.
- *Those Amazing Muscles Match Game.* A matching game format is used to teach anatomy.

- *NCLEX® Bingo.* Students study for NCLEX® using such categories as Name of disease, Complications, Labs, Examinations, and X-tras.
- *JCAHO Trivia.* This strategy develops agency-specific information to create a trivia quiz in preparation for a survey.
- *Collaboration Puzzle.* A puzzle format fosters team-building skills, commitment, shared vision, trust, and communication.
- *ABG Go Fish.* The traditional card game is used to teach blood gas interpretation; provides templates that may be copied from the book.
- *The Admission Shuffle.* Triage and admission skills are enhanced through use of a card game to make room assignments for pediatric admissions.

6. Dellinger, S: Communicating Beyond our Differences. Jade Ink, Tampa, FL, 1996.

   Description: This book teaches readers to assess their own personality type and to use the principles of geometric psychology to know themselves and work with others.

   Features: The book includes in-depth descriptions of the different personality types as symbolized by shapes (box, triangle, rectangle, circle, and squiggle) and describes how the different personalities behave at home, at work, and under stress. Implications for team work and "shape flexing" are included to enhance relationships and increase happiness and productivity.

Innovative Strategies:

- The positive and negative traits of each shape are examined.
- Suggestions help the reader work with people of each shape, including families, friends, spouses, and coworkers.
- Ideas for stress relief are included for each personality shape.
- The author discusses how shapes change across the life span.
- See **Shapes Define Your Personality** in this book.

7. DeYoung, S: Teaching Strategies for Nurse Educators. Prentice Hall, Upper Saddle River, NJ, 2003.

   Description: This comprehensive text includes much of the theoretical information nursing students need, as well as practical hints to enhance individual teaching styles.

   Features: Chapters discuss teaching and learning, assessing the learner, and using teaching strategies. Of the resources listed here, this book probably includes the greatest number of innovative strategies. The text also confronts issues, such as the multicultural aspects of learning, literacy and readability, and motivation and behavior change. Each chapter includes a case study, critical thinking exercises, and ideas for further research.

Innovative Strategies:
- *Imagery.* This method uses mental images to facilitate memorization of selected concepts.
- *Simulation Exercises.* This replication of a real situation calls for manipulation of selected variables—course of events, client condition changes, or situational details—to enhance learning and decision-making.
- *Self-learning Modules.* Packets are designed to let learners complete tasks at their own pace; each includes objectives, readings, and exercises.
- *Leveling of Questions.* Instructors consider the level of the questions they ask students orally, in assignments, and in testing. This strategy assesses levels of knowledge, understanding, and critical thinking.

8. Dunn, RS, and Griggs, SA: Learning Styles and the Nursing Profession. Jones and Bartlett, New York, 1998.
   Description: This unique book describes several frameworks for assessing diverse learning styles and adapting teaching methods to embrace them all.
   Features: The book examines the links between learning styles and teaching, the implications for educators in different settings, and a comparison between global and analytic thinkers. It includes several resources for further exploration of learning styles and teaching innovations. One chapter, *Eleven Steps Over the Brick Wall,* presents a step-by-step discussion of how to incorporate learning styles assessment and intervention methods into college and higher education curricula.

Innovative Strategies:
- *Task Cards.* Given questions and answers on separate cards, students match the cards as a study technique.
- *Flip Chute.* In this question-and-answer game, a card flips over while coming out of the question holder—made from a milk jug—and provides the answer.
- *Team Learning.* Group participants share the responsibility for answering questions and completing assignments.
- *Contract Activity Packages.* Objectives and topics are standard in this comprehensive learning strategy, but learners choose learning activities, resources, and reporting activities to complete the module. The essential component is the provision of alternative methods to accommodate the level of choice.

9. Fitzpatrick, J, and Montgomery, K: Career Strategies for Nurse Educators. F.A. Davis, Philadelphia, 2006.

Description: This unique book provides nurse educators with valuable tools for career success, hints for personal success, and survival techniques within the academic environment. It offers important information for those pursuing a career in nursing education, novice nursing instructors, and seasoned faculty.

Features: This book is divided into six sections: Personal Assessment, Your Curriculum Vitae, Preparing for the Interview, Surviving Your Initial Years as Faculty, Career Success Strategies for Clinical Faculty, and Success Strategies for Research Faculty. Each section presents strategies for meeting the challenges and opportunities associated with those tasks and career stages. Especially valuable are the tips solicited from many experienced nursing faculty and those in the "trenches" and new to nursing education.

Innovative Strategies:

- *Developing Your Teaching Dossier.* A template and hints help the nurse educator create a succinct but convincing curriculum vitae and dossier.
- *Understanding Academic Salary Structures.* Provides a basic guide to the compensatory frameworks common to academic environments.
- *Establishing a Publication Record.* Clarifies both the importance of and methods to create a record of publications and, if appropriate, a program of research.
- *Guidelines for Student Advisement.* General recommendations are given for student advisement in a variety of settings.
- *Gaining Certification in Nursing Education.* This section discusses the pros and con of, and the preparation for, attaining certification in nursing education.
- *Tips for Finding A Mentor.* This part gives basic advice for seeking out and maintaining a mentor in nursing education.
- *Using Networking to Advance Your Career and Career Satisfaction.* The personal and professional assets of networking with colleagues are discussed here.

10. Gaberson, K, and Oermann, MH: Clinical Teaching Strategies in Nursing. Springer, New York, 1999.

Description: This book provides a comprehensive set of information for new and experienced nursing instructors in the clinical area. Clinical instructors, who often are isolated from other instructors and learn through a "baptism by fire," will welcome this valuable resource. Many new instructors begin in the clinical area, and this book orients them to the role. Although designed for academic instructors, it may be valuable for clinical educators in the practice setting.

Features: Each chapter addresses a component of clinical teaching with information specific to nursing education. They encompass the range of clinical experiences, including supervised agency work, laboratories, simulations, conferences, observational experiences, use of preceptors, and self-directed learning activities. It also addresses clinical evaluation, competency assessment, and written assignments.

Innovative Strategies:

- *Use of Multimedia in Clinical Instruction.* This section guides instructors using multimedia tools in clinical instruction, and offers criteria for evaluating their usefulness in the clinical area.

- *Simulated Patients.* In this strategy, students use living "clients" to practice psychomotor and interpersonal communication skills.

- *Active Case Study.* Students analyze actual clinical cases. This skill sharpens decision-making and critical thinking skills.

- *Creating a Climate for Discussion.* Using these hints, instructors can create an atmosphere that encourages discussion and student contribution.

- *Concept Analysis Paper.* A written assignment explores concepts and applies them to clinical practice.

- *Teaching Plan.* This strategy details a client education project, including objectives, content, and teaching and evaluation strategies.

11. Glendon, KJ, and Ulrich, DL: Unfolding Case Studies: Experiencing the Realities of Clinical Nursing Practice. Prentice Hall, Upper Saddle River, NJ, 2001.

Description: This creative book provides many case studies requiring students to use critical thinking skills as a story unfolds. As more details come to the surface, students continue to problem-solve and use nursing knowledge to address issues.

Features: This book includes more than 60 exercises in pediatric, obstetrical, mental health, medical-surgical, and miscellaneous cases. Each case includes learning objectives, a story, focus questions, and a reflective writing exercise. Each case may have three to five parts that evolve through the course of the study, adding details and variables to the case. A workbook format allows students to write in their personal notes.

Innovative Strategies:

Unfolding Cases include:

- *Mandy and Amy—Student Nurses.* Confidentiality and nurse-client interactions are addressed.
- *Elsa Hunger.* Spiritual assessment and intervention are the focus of this study.
- *Joe Germaine.* This case examines the nursing care of a client with alcoholism.
- *Mary Martin.* The case of a Native American client with end-stage renal disease examines her nursing care and its cultural components.
- *Anna Rhodes.* This study focuses on vaginal bleeding and an emergency caesarian section.
- *Tracy Jones.* The nursing care of an infant with cleft lip and palate is described here.

12. Gross, R: Peak Learning: How to Create Your Own Lifelong Program for Personal Enlightenment and Professional Success. Putnam, New York, 1999.

   Description: This guidebook will enhance lifelong learning and growth. It deals with the use of technology, at-home exercises, workplace learning opportunities, distance education, and cognitive studies to enhance learning skills throughout an individual's life.

   Features: Self-help strategies and exercises enhance learning in others. Nurse educators will find several innovative strategies, along with learning and Web resources, information on the learning process, learning assessments, and strategies to enhance performance. Information about the author is available at www.adulted.about.com and www.RonaldGross.com.

Innovative Strategies:

- *The Six Thinking Hats.* See the **Six Hats Exercise** in this book. Gross suggests more ways to use this exercise for team building and decision-making.
- *Mind Mapping.* Similar to Concept Maps, these diagrams can represent concepts, processes, or class content.
- *Peak Learning Affirmations.* Positive statements guide personal learning.
- *Instant Replay.* Reexperiencing an encounter enhances and deepens the memory of it.

- *Pro-Active Reading.* The components of a book—cover, table of contents, introduction, preface, and index—are used to do a quick reading. See **Active Reading Conference** in this book.
- *Which are Your Strong Intelligences?, Your Best and Worst of Times,* and *Visualizing Your Learning Place.* Self-assessments are used to maximize learning potential.

13. Johnson, S, and Johnson, C: The One Minute Teacher: How to Teach Others to Teach Themselves. William Morrow/Quill, New York, 1986.

   Description: Part of the *One-Minute Manager Library,* this book provides a great inspiration to anyone who teaches. It reinforces our role as teachers to encourage and foster learning in others.

   Features: This enjoyable, quickly read book gives a positive feeling about collaborative learning. A clock becomes a visual cue to stimulate personal reflection. Exercises help readers learn to teach themselves and encourage that quality in others. The book is rich in quotations. A *One-Minute Teacher's Game Plan* captures the essence of its philosophy.

Innovative Strategies:

- *One-Minute Goal Setting.* Establish objectives and make sure behaviors match goals.
- *One-Minute Praising.* Every day, find something good about your performance or that of another and give it the recognition it deserves.
- *One-Minute Recovery.* Everyone needs to recover and learn from mistakes.

14. McKeachie, WJ, and Svinicki, M: McKeachie's Teaching Tips. Houghton Mifflin, Boston, 2006.

   Description: This book, designed for teachers in higher education, is an all-around resource for new instructors or those who need a refresher.

   Features: The book includes suggestions for course preparation, designing icebreakers, facilitating discussion, enhancing lectures, developing tests, and evaluating students. Interesting topics include dealing with cheating, teaching ethics, teachers as learners, teaching culturally diverse students, dealing with student problems, teaching in the laboratory, peer teaching, and motivation in the classroom. Each chapter includes a supplementary reading list and the text includes a comprehensive assembly of references.

Innovative Strategies:
- *Socratic Method.* The method of Socrates teaches by asking questions, encouraging thinking, and stimulating dialogue. Some may regard it as innovative.
- *Reading as Active Learning.* Hints for teachers and pointers for learners encourage students to get the most out of assigned readings.
- *Inner Circle.* Six to 15 students actively participate in the class and the rest serve as critical observers.
- *Teaching to Take Tests.* Students learn skills to help them demonstrate knowledge in a test format.
- *High-Stakes and Low-Stakes Writing.* This section suggests several class assignments and evaluation techniques.

15. Modly. DM, Zanotti, R, Poletti, P, and Fitzpatrick, J: Advancing Nursing Education Worldwide. Springer, New York, 1995.
    Description: This interesting book provides a global view of nursing education. It documents educational practices around the world, global issues confronting nursing education, and potential ways to advance nursing education through research and innovation.
    Features: Nurses from around the world share their thoughts on nursing education and address topics such as the teaching of nursing research and clinical judgment, trends in nursing education and healthcare, use of technology in education, teaching ethics, and socialization to the nursing profession.

Innovative Strategies:
- *Strategies to Advance Nursing Education Research.* Multiple strategies can increase the visibility, funding, and credibility of nursing education research.
- *Sister City Relationships.* These strategies build nursing education and research relationships between cities with economic and cultural ties.
- *Service Education Collaboration.* These guidelines promote the partnership between service and academics in preparing and maintaining nurses.
- *Guided Design.* In this problem-focused teaching method, students define problems, generate alternative solutions, and discuss responses.

16. Novotny, JM, and Quinn Griffin, MT: A Nuts-and-Bolts Approach to Teaching Nursing, ed 3. Springer, New York, 2006.
    Description: This is a general teaching guide for nursing faculty. It includes information on clinical teaching, classroom teaching, testing and evaluation, guiding students in

independent study, using technology, and helping students improve their writing skills.

Features: Each chapter includes instructions, tools, "nuts and bolts," and other helpful hints. The reader will find tables with explicit instructions, forms to guide teaching, and examples of note cards, group exercises, seminar guides, paper formats, and test hints.

Innovative Strategies:

- *Clinical Orientation.* This guide helps orient students to the clinical area.
- *Anecdotal Notes.* Guidelines suggest which information should be included in the documentation of student progress.
- *Contract Forms.* This section guides the instructor in establishing learning contracts with students.
- *Interpersonal Skills Rubric.* Group process and self-evaluation are assessed in a group exercise.
- *Textbook Evaluation Form.* This form provides criteria to use in assessing nursing education textbooks.
- *Checklist for Presentations.* Criteria are given for grading and evaluating student presentations.

17. Oermann, M, and Gaberson, K: Evaluation and Testing in Nursing Education. Springer, New York, 2005.

Description: This book provides a comprehensive look at evaluation, including testing, evaluating written assignments, clinical evaluation, and program evaluation. Developing valid and reliable exams; helping students prepare for licensure examinations; and social, ethical, and legal issues are among the topics addressed.

Features: This book offers a theory of evaluation, suggestions for test development, varieties of testing (fill-in-the-blank, multiple-choice, true-false, essay), evaluation of higher-order thinking (including critical thinking and problem-solving), examples of evaluation criteria, and helpful hints for new and experienced faculty. Each chapter has a summary and a reference list. The appendix includes clinical evaluation tools and other evaluation materials from several nursing education programs.

Innovative Strategies:

- *Code of Professional Responsibilities in Education Assessment.* This code was published by the National Council on Measurement in Education.
- *Code of Fair Testing Practice in Education.* This code was published by the Joint Committee on Testing Practices.

- *Examples of Rating Forms for Clinical Evaluation.* Formative and summative clinical evaluation tools from 15 nursing schools reflect associate degree to graduate nursing education evaluation.
- *Criteria for Evaluating Papers and Other Written Assignments.* This section suggests ways to assess content, organization, process, and writing style.
- *Percentage of Items in NCLEX®-RN Test Plan.* The blueprint for the NCLEX®-RN examination appears here.
- *Example of Analytic Scoring Rubric for Essay Items on Health-Care Issues.* This example of a grading rubric is adaptable for similar assignments.
- *Examples of Multiple-Choice Examination Questions.* Valid and invalid items demonstrate question construction techniques. See **In-class Test Questions** in this book.

18. Oermann, MH, and Heinrich, KT: Annual Review of Nursing Education, Volume 4. Springer, New York, 2006.
    Description: This yearly series, begun in 2003, combines the convenience of a book with the currency of a journal. Each review (there are currently four) addresses key issues confronting nursing education. The 20 chapters in each issue are essentially journal articles, including research studies, concept analyses, and descriptions of teaching challenges and solutions.
    Features: Each chapter deals with a selected topic: cooperative learning, teaching public policy, simulation laboratories, service learning, faculty development, the nursing student with ADHD, writing across the curriculum, the art of questioning, and many more.

Innovative Strategies:
- *Questioning.* Several pointers suggest ways to use questioning in clinical and didactic teaching environments. See **Clinical Questioning** in this book.
- *Using Handheld Technology.* Handheld personal digital assistants are discussed in relation to classroom and clinical teaching.
- *Numbered Heads.* Each student has a number. Instructor questions are directed toward individuals or groups as each number is called.
- *Participation Rubric.* This method evaluates classroom participation.
- *New Orientation CD-ROM.* This package for new students includes information essential to beginning a nursing program.
- *Grading for Asynchronous Online Discussions.* This chapter proposes a model for grading online discussion groups.

19. Rayfield, S, and Manning, L: Pathways of Teaching Nursing: Keeping it Real. ICAN Publishing, Bosier City, LA, 2006.

    Description: This compact book shares the insights of two experienced nurse educators and a philosophy of the teacher's role as the coach of an active learner. It incorporates the tenets of inspiration, engagement, relationships, empowerment, collaboration, and ownership in the teaching-learning process.

    Features: Each chapter addresses the basic tenets listed earlier and provides a description of strategies that reinforce each concept. The authors discuss their vast experiences with students and nursing education and provide inspiration for nurse educators to continually assess and modify their personal teaching styles.

Innovative Strategies:

- *Collaborative Testing* Three students work together to reach consensus on an examination. The students discuss and deliberate examination questions with each student handing in his or her own score sheet.

- *Using Illustrations to Create Visual Mnemonics.* The instructor creates or finds basic drawings to help students make mental associations. The text suggests several resources for obtaining these graphic, and sometimes amusing, depictions of nursing information.

- *Online Eternal Quiz.* Instructors provide an online quiz available "eternally" until the student is content with the achieved grade.

- *Student Surveys.* Students are polled about their perceptions related to coursework, general curriculum, and their course of study. The authors suggest an electronic medium for surveys in which students can reflect on learning, self-evaluation, and course evaluation.

- *Sounds into PowerPoint.* Sounds can be incorporated into slide presentations to provide a brief diversion from the lecture. They include breath sounds, heart sounds, different coughs, amusing jingles, and others.

- *Examination Blueprints.* These guidelines help to establish content validity in examinations and clinical reasoning tests.

20. Smith, MJ, and Fitzpatrick, JJ: Best Practices in Nursing Education: Stories of Exemplary Teachers. Springer, New York, 2006.

    Description: This compendium of stories profiles 23 exemplary teachers and provides their insights on teaching and learning.

    Features: Although written as an anthology of teachers' thoughts on best practices, the book includes many perspectives on innovation in teaching and learning from some of the premier nurse educators of our time. The chapters include each nurse educator's background, story introduction, early interest in teaching, preparation for teaching, mentoring for teaching, evolution as a teacher, feeling comfortable as a teacher, challenges, embarrassing teaching moments, most and least rewarding aspects of teaching, maintaining excellence as a teacher, and advice for new teachers. The final chapter includes teaching tips for a variety of nursing education venues.

Innovative Strategies:
- Tables include "Faculty Teaching Tips and Techniques," "Faculty Perspectives of What Does Not Work," "Student Perspectives," "Students Perspectives of What Teachers Do that Does Not Help Them Learn," and "Meaningful Advice Given to Teachers by Students."
- These tables are tailored to each of the following course types: didactic, clinical, distance education, and research.

21. Ulrich, DL, and Glendon, KJ: Interactive Group Learning: Strategies for Nurse Educators, ed. 2. Springer, New York, 2005.
    Description: This book provides the foundation for collaborative learning. It features a model for group learning, strategies to enhance group learning, and methods to use in group strategies.

    Features: Each chapter includes useful information on bringing collaborative teaching into the classroom. The authors describe their Comprehensive Group Learning Model. The book provides important information on group process and function and suggests ways to incorporate group interaction into many learning venues. Strategies and teaching hints make students feel comfortable and help them learn through creative teaching methods.

Innovative Strategies:
- *Fishbone.* In this strategy, replicated from the business world, students diagram a problem by considering multiple solutions.
- *Concept Case Analysis.* As in a case study, students select key data from a case to develop nursing interventions.
- *Tic-Tac Test Ready.* This version of Tic-Tac-Toe uses the popular game format for a test review.
- *Faculty/Student Drawing.* Faculty or students stimulate memories through drawings related to class material.

- *Let's Play Nurse.* Instructor-generated questions use NURSE®
  bingo cards to review for tests or prepare for NCLEX®.
- *Empathy Experiences.* As in **Day In the Life of a Client with . . .,**
  pairs of students try to replicate the challenges experienced with
  specified illnesses or disabilities.
- *Academic Controversy.* Students confront dilemmas by addressing
  both sides of the controversy. The focus is on critical thinking
  rather than resolution. See **In-class Debate** in this book.
- *You Have to Have a Heart.* In this decision-making exercise, several
  students prioritize to determine who should receive the transplant
  of a donor heart.

22. Valiga, TM, and Bruderle, ER: Using the Arts and Humanities
    to Teach Nursing. Springer, New York, 1997.
    Description: This book supplies nursing educators with the
    creative tools needed to enhance their teaching. Literature,
    poetry, television, film, sculpture, drama, children's literature,
    opera, photography, paintings, and music are used to enrich
    nursing education.
    Features: For each creative strategy described, examples are provid-
    ed to reinforce such concepts as assessment, caring, diversity,
    family dynamics, leadership, interpersonal communications,
    and professionalism.

Innovative Strategies:
- *Mozart's Magic Flute.* Opera is used to teach about sadness, suicide, gender principles, and class divisions.
- *All I Ever Needed to Know I Learned in Kindergarten.* This strategy
  uses a popular lay text to portray values, priorities, sharing, anger
  management, and balanced living.
- *The Little Engine That Could.* A popular children's book is used to
  teach encouragement, stamina, and determination.
- *In the Living Year by Mike and the Mechanic.* A song expresses a
  son's torment over his father's death.
- See **Film Clips** and **Read a Story** in this book.

23. Vance, C, and Olson, RK: The Mentoring Connection in
    Nursing. Springer, New York, 1998.
    Description: Although not an educational text, this book
    addresses a key issue in nursing education—mentoring. This
    classic text examines the mentor connection, perspectives on
    mentorship, the process and context of mentorship, and ways
    to expand the mentor connection.

Features: The book includes testimonies of nurses and their mentoring experiences, interviews, definitions of concepts, interviews with mentors and protégés, and international stories of mentoring. It gives us a down-to-earth view of mentoring and its role in education, leadership, and personal growth.

Innovative Strategies:

- *Commandments of Mentoring.* This section describes the tenets of the mentoring relationship.
- *Being a Mentor—Finding a Mentor.* Guidelines for these concepts are provided.
- *Maximizing the Role Of Protégé.* This section examines aspects of the protégé role.
- *Four Career Stages.* The mentor-protégé relationship is followed through a career progression.
- *Two Worlds of Mentoring: A New Paradigm.* This part presents a female model of mentoring.

24. Van Betten, P, and Moriarty, M: Nursing Illuminations: A Book of Days. Mosby, St. Louis, 2004.

    Description: This book is a unique anthology of stories about figures and events in nursing history.

    Features: The format follows the days of the year. A journal of nursing vignettes profiles individuals who contributed to health care or to the nursing profession. The 366 different stories accommodate readers who choose Leap Year to partake of this entertaining book! Although designed for private reading, the many inspiring stories can be used in the classroom and clinical areas.

Innovative Strategies:

The nurses described include:

- *Margaret Higgins Sanger (September 14).* She advocated for birth control rights and education and eventually founded Planned Parenthood.
- *Agnes Hannah Von Kurowski Stanfield (January 8).* A nurse in World War I, she was noted for her care of soldiers in Italy and France, including Ernest Hemingway. So impressed was Mr. Hemingway that he used her as the model for the nurse in his famous novel *A Farewell to Arms.*
- *Susan Walking Bear Yellowtail (February 11).* A Native American healer, she was appointed to the Public Health, Education, and

Welfare Board by President John F. Kennedy to promote the health of her people.

- *Sojourner Truth (February 12).* This famous abolitionist also worked as a Civil War nurse, teacher of nursing skills, and women's rights advocate.
- *Janet M. Geister (May 17).* Working with the Children's Bureau in 1918, she combated poor nutrition in children, especially in rural areas, by spearheading the "Save 100,000 Babies" campaign.
- *Mother Theresa (August 27).* This world-famous nun ministered to the sick, poor, dying, and discouraged around the world and received the Nobel Peace Prize.
- *Lavinia Lloyd Dock (February 25).* A suffragist, war protester, and political activist, she helped to raise nursing to a profession.
- See the book for complete stories and 359 more interesting nurses.
- See **Read a Story, Set the Stage,** and **Quotation Pauses** in this book.

25. Young, LE, and Paterson, B: Teaching Nursing: Developing a Student Centered Approach. Lippincott Williams, & Wilkins, Philadelphia, 2007.

   Description: This newly published text presents both theory and foundation to support a nursing education course and offers strategies for the practicing nursing educator. Conveying the philosophy that nursing education should be student-centered, it reinforces the active role of the learner in the educational process.

   Features: Chapters are separated into sections such as "Teaching Nursing: Theories and Concepts," "Methods and Approaches to Student-Centered Learning in Nursing," "Constructing Nursing Curricula: Challenges and Issues," "Student-Centered Teaching: Challenges and Issues for Faculty," and "Toward a New Future." Each chapter has learning activities, resources for educators, and a reference list to complement subject matter.

Innovative Strategies:

- *Enlisting Narrative and Story as Ethics Teaching Strategies.* The use of stories increases the "realness" of ethical conflicts and stimulates personal thinking and deliberation. See **Read a Story** in this book.
- *McGill Model of Nursing.* This method teaches a client-centered approach to all nurses, and provides assessments and teaching strategies for the nursing education setting.

- *One Minute Question and Answer.* Instructors pose a question and give students 1 minute to consider potential answers. Students report back, and instructors provide feedback and discussion. See **One-Minute Class** in this book.
- *Preceptorship Pathways.* This section describes a method of clinical instruction for senior nursing students.
- *Criteria for Online Discussion Participation.* Specific parameters that can be used to evaluate performance in online discussions will be evaluated. See **Online Discussion Groups** in this book.

Strategy Locator

Index